Health, Disability and the Capability Approach

This book focuses on two areas of substantial and growing importance to the human development and capability approach: health and disability. The research on disability, health and the capability approach has been diverse in the topics it covers, and the conceptual frameworks and methodologies it uses, beginning over a decade and a half ago in health and more than a decade ago in disability. This book shares a set of contributions in these two areas: the first set of chapters focusing on disability; and the second set focusing on health and the health capability paradigm in particular.

This book was originally published as a special issue of the *Journal of Human Development and Capabilities.*

Sophie Mitra is Professor in the Department of Economics at Fordham University, New York City, USA. Her research interests centre on development economics, disability and applied microeconomics. She is co-editor of the Palgrave Studies in Disability and International Development series, and is also a fellow of the Human Development and Capability Association and a senior research associate at the Center for International Policy Studies.

Jennifer Prah Ruger is the Amartya Sen Professor of Health Equity, Economics and Policy at the University of Pennsylvania's School of Social Policy and Practice, and the Perelman School of Medicine. She is also the Director of the Master of Science in Social Policy Program, inaugural Associate Dean for Global Studies, and Faculty Chair at the Center for High Impact Philanthropy.

Health, Disability and the Capability Approach

Edited by
Sophie Mitra and Jennifer Prah Ruger

Routledge
Taylor & Francis Group
LONDON AND NEW YORK

First published 2018
by Routledge
2 Park Square, Milton Park, Abingdon, Oxon, OX14 4RN, UK

and by Routledge
711 Third Avenue, New York, NY 10017, USA

Routledge is an imprint of the Taylor & Francis Group, an informa business

British Library Cataloguing in Publication Data
A catalogue record for this book is available from the British Library

ISBN 13: 978-1-138-63490-9

Typeset in Times New Roman
by RefineCatch Limited, Bungay, Suffolk

Publisher's Note
The publisher accepts responsibility for any inconsistencies that may have arisen during the conversion of this book from journal articles to book chapters, namely the possible inclusion of journal terminology.

Contents

	Citation Information	vii
	Notes on Contributors	ix
	Health, Disability and the Capability Approach: An Introduction *Jennifer Prah Ruger & Sophie Mitra*	1
1.	An Analysis of the Intentions of a Chilean Disability Policy Through the Lens of the Capability Approach *Alvaro Díaz Ruiz, Natalia Sánchez Durán & Alexis Palá*	11
2.	Towards a Disability-inclusive Higher Education Policy through the Capabilities Approach *Oliver Mutanga & Melanie Walker*	29
3.	Disability and Poverty in Morocco and Tunisia: A Multidimensional Approach *Jean-Francois Trani, Parul Bakhshi, Sarah Myers Tlapek, Dominique Lopez & Fiona Gall*	46
4.	Corporate Contributions to Developing Health Capabilities *Regina Moczadlo, Harald Strotmann & Jürgen Volkert*	76
5.	India, Health Inequities, and a Fair Healthcare Provision: A Perspective from Health Capability *Rhyddhi Chakraborty & Chhanda Chakraborti*	94
6.	Health Economics and Ethics and the Health Capability Paradigm *Jennifer Prah Ruger*	108
7.	Exploring Different Interpretations of the Capability Approach in a Health Care Context: Where Next? *Philip Kinghorn*	127
	Index	145

Citation Information

The chapters in this book were originally published in the *Journal of Human Development and Capabilities*, volume 16, issue 4 (November 2015). When citing this material, please use the original page numbering for each article, as follows:

Introduction

Health, Disability and the Capability Approach: An Introduction
Jennifer Prah Ruger & Sophie Mitra
Journal of Human Development and Capabilities, volume 16, issue 4 (November 2015), pp. 473–482

Chapter 1

An Analysis of the Intentions of a Chilean Disability Policy Through the Lens of the Capability Approach
Alvaro Díaz Ruiz, Natalia Sánchez Durán & Alexis Palá
Journal of Human Development and Capabilities, volume 16, issue 4 (November 2015), pp. 483–500

Chapter 2

Towards a Disability-inclusive Higher Education Policy through the Capabilities Approach
Oliver Mutanga & Melanie Walker
Journal of Human Development and Capabilities, volume 16, issue 4 (November 2015), pp. 501–517

Chapter 3

Disability and Poverty in Morocco and Tunisia: A Multidimensional Approach
Jean-Francois Trani, Parul Bakhshi, Sarah Myers Tlapek, Dominique Lopez & Fiona Gall
Journal of Human Development and Capabilities, volume 16, issue 4 (November 2015), pp. 518–548

Chapter 4

Corporate Contributions to Developing Health Capabilities
Regina Moczadlo, Harald Strotmann & Jürgen Volkert
Journal of Human Development and Capabilities, volume 16, issue 4 (November 2015), pp. 549–566

Chapter 5

India, Health Inequities, and a Fair Healthcare Provision: A Perspective from Health Capability
Rhyddhi Chakraborty & Chhanda Chakraborti
Journal of Human Development and Capabilities, volume 16, issue 4 (November 2015), pp. 567–580

Chapter 6

Health Economics and Ethics and the Health Capability Paradigm
Jennifer Prah Ruger
Journal of Human Development and Capabilities, volume 16, issue 4 (November 2015), pp. 581–599

Chapter 7

Exploring Different Interpretations of the Capability Approach in a Health Care Context: Where Next?
Philip Kinghorn
Journal of Human Development and Capabilities, volume 16, issue 4 (November 2015), pp. 600–616

Notes on Contributors

Parul Bakhshi is Assistant Professor in the Occupational Therapy Program at Washington University, St Louis, USA. She has been carrying out research in low-income countries for the last 10 years, working on issues linked to international development. She is currently working on stigma and social exclusion of destitute groups that impede participation within society.

Chhanda Chakraborti is Professor of Philosophy in the Department of Humanities and Social Sciences, Indian Institute of Technology Kharagpur, India. Her active research interests include bioethics and public health ethics, as well as the philosophy of mind. She holds a PhD from the University of Utah, USA.

Rhyddhi Chakraborty holds a PhD from the Indian Institute of Technology Kharagpur, India. Her research has an interest in applied ethics (especially bioethics), infectious disease ethics and environmental ethics. Her current research interest is in the philosophical social justice theory of health capability.

Alvaro Díaz Ruiz is Professor of Public Health Administration and Health Management at the University San Sebastian, Santiago, Chile. He is currently a doctoral candidate in Management and Public Policy at the National University of Cordoba, Colombia. He is also Director of the Equalitas Foundation.

Fiona Gall is the Director of the Agency Coordinating Body of Afghan Relief and Development. She has extensive experience in humanitarian and development programs focusing on disability and gender particularly in Pakistan and Afghanistan. She led Sandy Gall Appeal for Afghanistan for 10 years and specialized in community-based rehabilitation programs.

Philip Kinghorn is a Research Fellow in the Institute of Applied Health Research, University of Birmingham, UK. His research concerns conceptual frameworks and methodology for the economic evaluation of health and social care interventions. He works on projects which have used the capability approach to conceptualize patients' experiences of receiving health care and to evaluate care at the end of life.

Dominique Lopez is an independent researcher whose work focuses on health issues such as drug use, disability and reproductive health. Her recent professional experience provides her with an extra dimension in understanding heterogeneous data collection systems, as well as confidence in the negotiation and collaboration with scientific working groups or liaising a certain policy and decision-making levels.

Sophie Mitra is Professor in the Department of Economics at Fordham University, New York City, USA. Her research interests centre on development economics, disability and applied microeconomics. She is co-editor of the Palgrave Studies in Disability and

International Development series, and is also a Fellow of the Human Development and Capability Association and a Senior Research Associate at the Center for International Policy Studies.

Regina Moczadlo is Professor of Economics at the Hochschule Pforzheim, Germany. Her research focus lies in international economics and foreign direct investments. She was previously Director of the Department for Business Formation and Continued Training at the Chamber of Industry and Commerce Rhein-Neckar, Mannheim.

Oliver Mutanga is Marie Curie Scientia Research Fellow in the Department of Community Medicine and Global Health at the University of Oslo, Norway, where his research is based around health and disability. He holds a PhD from the University of the Free State, South Africa.

Alexis Palá holds a Bachelor's Degree in Anthropology from the University of Notre Dame, USA. She conducted her undergraduate fieldwork in Santiago, Chile and Madrid, Spain on societal perceptions of adults with intellectual disabilities and the opportunities afforded to them. She is currently undertaking fieldwork in Chile as a Fulbright Scholar.

Jennifer Prah Ruger is the Amartya Sen Professor of Health Equity, Economics and Policy at the University of Pennsylvania's School of Social Policy and Practice, and the Perelman School of Medicine. She is also the Director of the Master of Science in Social Policy Program, inaugural Associate Dean for Global Studies, and Faculty Chair at the Center for High Impact Philanthropy.

Natalia Sánchez Durán is the Vice President of the SientoporCiento Foundation, a day center for people with severe intellectual disability. She holds a Master's Degree in Public Policy from the University of Chile, Santiago, Chile.

Harald Strotmann is Professor of Economics at the Hochschule Pforzheim, Germany. He has led many research projects, including an evaluation of German labor market reforms, and several projects contributing to the Poverty and Wealth Report. His research focuses on microdata analyses and questions of the labor market and social policy.

Sarah Myers Tlapek is Assistant Professor in the School of Social Work at the University of Missouri, USA. Her research focuses on the relationships between trauma, mental health and interpersonal violence, and she is particularly interested in examining ways that exposure to one type of violence may increase the risk for future interpersonal violence.

Jean-Francois Trani is Assistant Professor in the Brown School of Social Work at Washington University, St Louis, USA. His work lies at the intersection of mental health, disability, vulnerability and poverty with a focus on conducting research that informs policy and service design for individuals living in conflict affected and low-income states.

Jürgen Volkert is Professor of Economics at Hochschule Pforzheim, Germany. He is a member of the scientific advisory board of the German government for official poverty and wealth reporting. His research and publications focus on the capability approach, poverty and ethics, as well as on sustainable human development and its main actors and determinants.

Melanie Walker is currently the Vice President of the Human Development and Capability Association, and a Senior Research Professor at the University of the Free State, South Africa, where she is Director of the Centre for Research on Higher Education and Development.

Health, Disability and the Capability Approach: An Introduction†

JENNIFER PRAH RUGER & SOPHIE MITRA

This special issue of the *Journal of Human Development and Capabilities* focuses on two areas of substantial and growing importance to the human development and capability approach: disability and health. The research on disability, health and the capability approach has been diverse in the topics it covers, and the conceptual frameworks and methodologies it uses, beginning over a decade and a half ago in health (Ruger 1998) and more than a decade ago in disability (Baylies 2002).[1] We are pleased to share a set of articles in these two areas. The first set of articles focuses on disability, while the second set of articles focuses on health and the health capability paradigm (HCP), in particular.

Disability

This special issue starts with three articles on disability. Disability has figured in a number of the writings of both Martha Nussbaum and Amartya Sen (e.g. Nussbaum 2006; Sen 2009a). For example, Sen has used disability in numerous examples while exposing the capability approach (e.g. Sen 1985, 5). Later, Sen stressed the relevance of disability "for the understanding of deprivation in the world" and as "one of the most important arguments for paying attention to the capability perspective" (Sen 2009b, 258). Starting more than a decade ago, the capability approach has been used by other scholars in different disciplines to study various disability issues. For instance, it has been used to consider the relationship between disability and human development (Baylies 2002). It has been used to conceptualize disability in general as capability deprivation among persons with impairments (e.g. Burchardt 2004; Mitra 2006) or in specific contexts, such as education (Terzi 2005) or public policy (Trani et al. 2011). It has also been used to analyze the economic well-being of persons with disabilities, especially with respect to what Sen calls the "earnings handicap" and the "conversion handicap" experienced by persons with disabilities (e.g.

†Ruger was guest editor on health and wrote the introduction section on health. Mitra was guest editor on disability and wrote the introduction section on disability.

Kuklys 2005). The literature at the intersection of the capability approach and disability has grown since and continues to grow, as shown by the disability articles in this special issue.

The Diaz et al. (2015) article analyzes the intentions of a disability policy in Chile. In recent years, increasing emphasis has been placed on program evaluations in development for purposes of learning or accountability by various stakeholders (international organizations, national actors, and donors). The stress has been placed on impact evaluations, and in some disciplines, certain methodologies have become dominant such as randomized controlled trials in development economics. The Diaz et al. article conducts an evaluation of a different kind, nonetheless ripe with insights. It focuses on the intentions of a disability program: the Ministry of Health's home-based care program for persons with severe disabilities aged 65 years and above. The idea is simple: if the intentions of the program are not in line with enhancing justice as per the capability approach, then the program in practice is unlikely to improve the situation of this group and is in need for reform. The authors conduct a content analysis of the official text of the program on underlying intentions of achievement, agency, freedom and well-being. They find that the program's intentions fall short on all accounts, and especially with respect to agency and freedom. This important finding makes us want to ask: Are the intentions of other disability programs in Chile and elsewhere also not justice-enhancing? This could be found by conducting similar studies for other disability programs, run by government or non-governmental organizations. Of course, such an analysis could be applied to policies beyond disability, including in health and poverty reduction. This article shows that, with relatively limited resources, content analysis can provide insights to uncover policies and programs that, in their intentions, do not enhance justice and therefore need reforms. It is thus a useful tool in the researcher and policy analyst's toolbox.

The Mutanga and Walker (2015) article analyzes the capabilities of students with disabilities in higher education in South Africa. While the rights to education for persons with disabilities is recognized under the 2006 United Nations Convention on the Rights of Persons with Disabilities (Article 24), students with disabilities continue to face serious challenges accessing schools or in schools. Efforts to make education more inclusive are hampered by a lack of data and research on these challenges and how to solve them. Mutanga and Walker contribute to fill this gap in the literature by collecting qualitative data from students with disabilities in two universities in South Africa. They identify 11 capabilities valued by the students: aspiration, cultural value, choice of identity, educational resilience, knowledge and imagination, language, mobility, religious affiliation, respect dignity and recognition, social relation and social networks, and voice. Students with disabilities often report lacking these capabilities, so the authors show for students with disabilities, the gap between their lived experiences and what they value in higher education. Their deprivations and valued capabilities have implications for policy. Education policy outcomes typically focus on few quantifiable achievements such as student graduation rates and exam performance. Yet, this study shows that the capabilities students with disabilities value and the deprivations they face are broad and multifaceted. The authors argue that these capabilities valued by students with disabilities can be secured by embedding them in curriculum and in higher education institutions. The authors find that individual agency and choice is important in these students' lives. They conclude that this highlights a contribution of the capability approach compared to other disability models, in that it places individual agency at the center stage.

The Trani et al. (2015) article is a study of multidimensional poverty and disability for Morocco and Tunisia. Unlike earlier such studies in low- and middle-income countries (Mitra, Posarac, and Vick 2013; Trani and Cunnings 2013), the authors have data for all age groups and measure functionings in a wide range of dimensions. They find a significant association between disability and multidimensional poverty and thus demonstrate the need to include disability in poverty reduction policy, research, and data collection. Studies on multidimensional poverty have multiplied in recent years. The Multidimensional Poverty Index (MPI) (Alkire and Santos 2014), based on the capability approach, is increasingly used in research and policy. In brief, it is a measure of the experience of simultaneous multiple deprivations for households. This article offers a complementary way of implementing a multidimensional poverty analysis in that it uses the individual as a unit of analysis, compared to the household in the MPI. This is suitable for the analysis of potential patterns of disadvantage based on individual characteristics, such as age, sex, and disability status. As a matter of fact, the authors end up finding that persons with disabilities, and especially women with disabilities, are more likely to experience multiple deprivations than persons without disabilities. Such an analysis therefore shows the need for complementary analysis of multidimensional poverty at the individual level. Overall, this article offers the type of comparative assessments that, Sen argues, are essential to develop justice-enhancing reforms (2009a, 401).

Together, these articles, framed in the context of the capability approach, highlight the importance of disability in human development. They show that if development policies are going to positively impact the lives of persons with disabilities, these policies need to enhance the capabilities of persons with disabilities in a wide range of dimensions, including education (Mutanga et al. 2015), health-care services (Diaz et al. 2015), employment, social participation, psychological well-being and physical safety (Trani et al. 2015). Broadly, these articles have implications for assessing capabilities and public policies in human development in general, and for persons with disabilities and other groups, in particular.[2]

Health

The health articles address a number of themes at the intersection of health and capability.

The article by Moczadlo et al. (2015) focuses on an important and understudied pillar—the private sector—of the health economy. In the transition from international to global health, the dominance of United Nations agencies and bilateral arrangements has been replaced with a greater focus on private sector development and public–private partnerships. The contemporary global health architecture consists of a plurality of global and domestic health actors, many of which stem from private entities. Some of this transformation has been spurred by government failures and some by advances in technology and science, couched in the recognition that narrow medical interventions are inadequate to the challenge of the social and economic determinants of health. And in terms of human development, a corporation's investment in its employees and consumers' well-being has benefits that accrue in the short and long term, both for companies and for society overall. While a healthier and more productive workforce and clientele mean a greater return on investment for companies, the enhancement of individuals' substantive freedoms benefits all. The resources, innovation, and expertise that corporations can bring to global health is auspicious, for example, Merck & Company, Inc., helped control and eliminate river blindness in affected regions through the donation of Mectizan. Can the distribution networks and supply chain systems of Coca-Cola, for example, be leveraged to deliver condoms or oral rehydration therapy? Despite this promise, more often than not, multilateral corporations succumb to short-term inducements from investors over long-term improvement of societal well-being. Who then holds the private sector accountable?

It is in this context that the article by Moczadlo et al. invites our attention on assessing the corporate impacts on capabilities and sustainable human development. In independently evaluating health initiatives in the Bayer CropScience's Model Village Project (MVP) this study estimates both the corporate potential and risks. Through a mixed-methods analysis, employing both quantitative and qualitative techniques, of two model and two control villages, researchers concentrate on health and health capabilities and offer results on trust, a vital ingredient to understanding both the process and outcomes of sustainable human development. A key distinction between subjective health perceptions and objective health and nutrition is made and data are collected and analyzed to better understand this gap. Trust is described by the authors as depending upon positive expectations about an individual or organization's motivation or behavior that allows a person to be vulnerable to that entity's actions. Corporate health initiatives, in this context, are seen as "corporate benevolence" that creates the kind of positive experience required to build trust in the asymmetric business relationship between multinational corporations and individuals, in this case farmers, in resource-constrained settings. The asymmetry in resources and power are important dimensions of the context within which private sector organizations either facilitate or thwart capability expansion.

In their results, Moczadlo et al. found a gap between subjective health perceptions and objective health status, demonstrating a significant lack of health awareness, possibly reflecting adaptation, apathy, and insufficient health knowledge. This was particularly acute in assessments of food quality and intake and malnutrition. Malnutrition is one of the most vexing health problems in India, where 39% of Indian children are stunted and 42% of Indian women are underweight before pregnancy due to poor nutrition. Villagers also indicated that health was one of the most important dimensions of their well-being and underscored health agency and responsibility. Half of the population distrusted multinational corporations.

Among the Bayer CropScience initiatives, the health camps served over 850 people, primarily diagnosing the difference between the objective health situation and subjective health perceptions. The water purification plant installation and dissemination had mixed results due to a lack of awareness of the benefits of purified water, and the dental camp treated children who had major dental problems and all children received tooth paste and a tooth brush and planned check-ups every six months. These activities improved villagers' access to health care and to health risk mitigation; the majority of participants saw improvements in their well-being as a result of the health-related activities. There are risks, however, that corporate strategies neglect significant parts of the population and do not replace the role of a strong and reliable public sector. This study underscores the important differentiation between health capabilities and health preferences (affected by habits, traditions, culture, and accepted customs).

The article by Chakraborty et al. (2015) focuses on the health system as a major institution in a health society. This article fits well with the global and national movement for universal health coverage as a sustainable development goal. The post-2015 development agenda is focused on well-being for all and universal health coverage in terms of health promotion, prevention, treatment, and financial risk protection. In their article, Chakraborty et al. analyze the Indian health-care system from a health capability perspective and argue that to address health inequalities, the Indian health-care system should reform the vision of health underlying the national health policy, focus on delivering health services to all, and employ key concepts of the HCP as guiding principles for providing universal health coverage.

Health inequalities in India vary across social and economic groups, yet characteristics of the public health-care system contribute to inequities in the HCP central health capabilities, the capability to avoid escapable diseases and premature death. Many limiting factors of the health-care system exist that include low public health disbursements (4% of GDP) and very high out of pocket health-care expenditures, both of which create vulnerabilities and insecurities among the population. Additionally, applying the HCP concept of shortfall sufficiency, the allocation, and capacity of health resources in India exhibits a significant underperformance, making it impossible for all to access necessary and appropriate care. Finally, human resources for health are significantly compromised, large proportions of health positions are vacant and rural populations, in particular, lack sufficient information and well-trained and equipped expert personnel and diagnostic and treatment equipment and facilities. Health system deficiencies affect groups' and individuals' actual and potential health.

In order to address these social problems, Chakraborty et al. propose a social justice framework based on the HCP as the basis for public policy for health in India. The authors advance the principle of special moral importance for health capability. With a focus on the central health capabilities, the Indian framework emphasizes the freedom to achieve health functionings and health agency, the ability of the group or individual to pursue valuable health goals. Even if society guarantees equal access to high-quality medically necessary and appropriate health care, individuals must exercise their health agency to translate these resources into good health. The authors argue that the public health-care system and individuals have a shared obligation to create conditions where all can exercise health agency and effectuate health capability and they are especially concerned about individuals' exposure to risk and their ability to adequately manage it. They provide a vision to guide the health system reform in India and policy recommendations for addressing health inequalities.

The next article by Ruger (2015) advances a new interdisciplinary field of study, health capability economics. Health capability economics combines theory and research methods from ethics and economics, using a combination of concepts and techniques from these fields in order to avoid the deficiencies that result from a single-perspective approach. In neoclassical health economics, expected utility, strict rationality, and consumer theory are still used despite their limitations in explanatory power and in providing guiding principles for difficult social problems. The same is true for welfare health economics, which, despite a shift from the microeconomic tools of supply and demand analysis based in consumer theory to the use of the social welfare function to select the "best" social option, is limited in its ability to explain the behavior of individuals and institutions in relation to health, particularly the role of equity and need. While extra-welfarist analysis was an effective move away from both neoclassical and welfare health economics by incorporating non-welfarist evaluations, such as health in its calculations, extra-welfarism, too, falls short of explaining human behavior and developing guiding principles for public policy, particularly collective choice grounded in social justice. On the ethics side, bioethics and medical ethics, have failed to fully consider opportunity costs and cost functions, efficiency, uncertainty and risk, asymmetric information and other market failures, and health production and health system reform.

Health capability economics emerges to account for these incongruities by integrating ethical and economic factors in understanding individual and societal health decision-making. A predominant issue in health capability economics involves understanding several strata of individual and collective choice in health and health-care. One branch relates to recognizing the major deviations from the conditions of perfect competition – and thus the falsity of the First and Second Theorems of Welfare Economics—of the health and health-care sectors—concerned particularly with uncertainty, information, public goods, and externalities. Economists would argue that violations of the principles of Pareto efficiency and competitive markets put us in a second best world where the best social scientific theory and methods (economic) are compromised. But the Pareto principle does not include important ethical values, for example, distributional concerns, nor is it necessarily based on people's interests, which can diverge from their preferences (Fleurbaey 2007).

Health capability economics takes a different tack, highlighting three prevalent themes: need, equity, and efficiency. It conveys normative judgments about the fairness of markets for health and health-care and what the goals of health policy and public policy for health ought to be. Health capability economics does not, however, eschew positive economics rather this interdisciplinary field re-orientates positive economics toward the empirical consequences of policies focused on ethically important issues that have normative conclusions. It analyzes—and the founding branch of it advances a particular view of—the normative foundations of criteria for comparing advantage and disadvantage and their distribution across society. What is a fair way in which to allocate resources? How would changes in health policy and health system reform impact health equity? How can equitable public policies affecting health be implemented? What are the implications of public moral norms of equity in health for collective choice and social organization? How should the worst-off be treated by society?

The HCP is the founding branch of health capability economics. The HCP has sought a thorough understanding of the properties of a health society, of ethical principles and empirical methods (quantitative and qualitative) and the allocation of resources in terms of health equity criteria. Its focus has been on individuals' health capabilities in terms of their health functioning, health agency, and health needs. The HCP cross-fertilizes between ethics and economics; a focus on health equity and the shortfall sufficiency principle including priority to the worst-off; justifying a theory of fair allocation in terms of equality in health capabilities as an intrinsically and instrumentally valued component of the capability set. The HCP rejects incommensurable health preferences and utilities and their interpersonal comparisons across individuals and shifts the focus from resources and liberties to capabilities and functionings. The HCP seeks individual achievement and the freedom for achievement, along with equality in capability sets, sets of functionings accessible to individuals, and their health agency. By focusing on capabilities rather than achievements alone, the HCP accounts for both individual and societal responsibility for health equity.

Health capability economics focuses on criteria for evaluating social states and social policies, both at the individual and societal levels. The HCP holds that personal preferences about health and health-care should not be the basis for rank ordering social states, rather individuals' well-considered interests should be the indicator. The HCP provides better resources than neoclassical or standard welfare health economics or extra-welfarism, for normatively grasping individual vis-à-vis social responsibility. At the same time, the HCP incorporates positive economic methods of empirically examining the consequences of policy choices and integrates procedures and consequences in describing and evaluating social states. It broadens the analysis scope beyond the narrow consequentialism found in neoclassical and standard welfare health economics and extra-welfarism. Through a multi-stage process drawing on insights from ethics, economics, and public health and medical sciences, the HCP offers a way out of the dilemma of providing a small gain to many individuals at the cost of providing a large gain to a person who is badly off and of the dilemma of providing a small gain to the worst-off with exorbitant costs to society and losses in the central health capabilities of others. The HCP also weakens the neoclassical assumption of perfect selfishness in cooperation and social choice and includes studies of fairness, altruism, and inequity aversion.

Starting about a decade and a half ago, capability theory began to be applied to health and health-care (Ruger 1998; Sen 2009b) and subsequent interpretations of the capability approach have emerged in this growing field of theoretical and empirical scholarship. The article by Kinghorn (2015) takes stock of four applications of the capability approach to health and health-care: the HCP, the OCAP/OxCAP instruments (Lorgelly et al. 2008), ICECAP instruments (Coast et al. 2008), and the assessment of patients with chronic pain. (Kinghorn 2010) The article then discusses a possible path, including issues to be addressed, for future research in this field in the future. The article identifies two key motivations in this field: (1) facilitating agreement on a core concept of health and (2) capability as an alternative to utilitarian health maximization. Kinghorn argues that extra-welfarism, using the Quality-Adjusted-Life-Year (QALY), is an alternative to a strict welfarist approach, but does not constitute an application of the capability approach due to its focus on health maximization and exclusion of capabilities and equity. The article analyzes these four strands in the field in terms, respectively, of the capability set, valuing objects within the capability set, and decision-making.

The scope of and methods used to define the capability set differs across the four approaches. The OCAP/OxCAP instruments (Lorgelly et al. 2008) refine an existing survey, from the British Household Panel Survey based on Nussbaum's 10 central capabilities. Some questions are phrased in terms of functionings while others ask about ability, all are combined into an index of 18 questions. The ICECAP instruments (Coast et al. 2008) are used for different populations: older people, the general adult population (Al-Janabi, Flynn, and Coast 2012), and supportive care at the end of life. The patients with chronic pain assessment (Kinghorn 2010) is participatory and focuses on identifying capabilities important to patients with chronic pain. It has been developed into a questionnaire for such patients. The HCP focuses on two central health capabilities (Ruger 2004). Quantitative research has been conducted with this approach to understand the impact of health insurance reforms, the effect of health expenses on household capabilities and coping mechanism among poor households in Vietnam (Nguyen et al. 2012a, 2012b, 2012c). Health agency has been studied qualitatively in India (Feldman et al. 2015).

Kinghorn (2015) also compares and contrasts the different approaches in valuing objects in the capability set. For example, for the OxCAP-MH (Simon, Anand et al. 2013), equal weights were assigned to each dimension, combined into an index, and for the ICECAP instruments best–worst scaling is used, whereas researchers and policy-makers can employ the health capability profile with scales and subscales (Ruger 2010). Health capability profile constructs have been developed for studies in Vietnam, and empirical health systems and medical research in low- and middle-income countries have employed the HCP. Central health capabilities can be determined through a process of incompletely theorized agreements with priority for central, above non-central, health capabilities. Like the HCP before, the ICECAP constitutes life as a prerequisite for other capabilities and thus absence of life is equal to absence of capability. The chronic pain instrument treats physical and mental well-being as a central capability such that the overall well-being score is reduced to zero where no capability exists in these dimensions.

For decision-making, the article argues that the ICECAP (Coast et al. 2008) uses preference-type information to create a common index and completely ordered states, while the chronic pain instrument (Kinghorn 2010) explores relative values but does not provide a general rule. The HCP advances shortfall sufficiency to determine need and priority for which a partial ordering of health capabilities or health functionings is what is required for analysis. A minimal threshold, as a minimum obligation to society, sets a constraint on redistribution. In the HCP, efficiency is also an important consideration in addition to equity; resources are used efficiently toward those in need as opposed to increasing the greatest general overall societal welfare. Applications of the HCP have conducted empirical and ethical work on adult and child mortality, employing cluster analytical techniques, to establish a global norm or threshold of achievable health (Ruger and Kim 2006; Ruger 2006). Adopting shortfall sufficiency with equity and efficiency criteria would result in substantial policy and research shifts as compared to other allocation schemes. For example, the HCP would prioritize areas such as rare diseases with a smaller demographic but a greater share of resources. The article endorses shortfall sufficiency and gives it "monopoly-like status" because the author argues that it is the only suggestion found in the four approaches.

Kinghorn (2015) then goes on to discuss the implications of taking health as the sole objective for analysis as compared with, or even in addition to, evaluating health within the broader capability set. The HCP addresses this empirically and theoretically with health capabilities as part of the broader set of capabilities in allocating resources and extends beyond the QALY metric to include the ability to pursue health as well as health outcomes. The HCP also extends the determinants and sectors influencing health beyond health care alone. The HCP and extra-welfarism share the position that health deprivations below the threshold cannot be compensated by expansions elsewhere in the capability set and the HCP identifies the intrinsic and interrelated importance of health capabilities. By contrast, the ICECAP-O/A has no dimensions directly related to health and would need to be used in conjunction with a health-related instrument. From the ICECAP-O/A perspective the relevant endpoint is a broad concept of well-being. The patient with chronic pain assessment includes measures related to life expectancy and attention-seeking symptoms, such as physical discomfort, pain, and depression. For the patients with chronic pain assessment, both symptoms and broader well-being are important. While directly assessing capability is not possible, research on health agency focused on "perceived abilities" as well as "abilities", whereas other approaches have attempted to ask people about their functioning levels and their freedoms to function in terms of self-reported functionings and self-perceived capability.

The articles in this special issue on disability and health all attempt to develop or apply conceptual frameworks related to the capability approach to develop better policies and assess their impacts. While these articles are not necessarily representative of the scholarship on disability and health through the lens of the capability approach, they show part of a diverse and rich body of research that has been developing in these areas.

Disclosure statement

No potential conflict of interest was reported by the authors.

Notes

1. The bibliography published as an online addendum to this issue provides a compendium of works on health, disability and the capability approach.
2. It should be noted that the health articles in this issue are not unrelated to disability and may well have implications for the analysis of disability issues through the capability approach. For instance, the Health Capability Paradigm and its consideration of needs is pertinent to the analysis of the conversion handicap mentioned above. In addition, the three interpretations of the capability approach in a health-care context that focus on assessing well-being overall (OCAP/OxCAP, ICECAP, chronic pain assessment), as reviewed in the article by Kinghorn, can be considered as assessments of disability conceptualized as capability deprivation among persons with impairments or health conditions (Burchardt 2004; Mitra 2006, Forthcoming).

References

Al-Janabi, H., T. Flynn, and J. Coast. 2012. "Development of a Self-Report Measure of Capability Wellbeing for Adults: The ICECAP-A." *Quality of Life Research* 21 (1): 167–176.

Alkire, S., and M. E. Santos. 2014. "Measuring Acute Poverty in the Developing World: Robustness and Scope of the Multidimensional Poverty Index." *World Development* 59: 251–274.

Baylies, C. 2002. "Disability and the Notion of Human Development: Questions of Rights and Capabilities." *Disability & Society* 17 (7): 725–739.

Burchardt, T. 2004. "Capabilities and Disability: The Capabilities Framework and the Social Model of Disability." *Disability & Society* 19 (7): 735–751.

Chakraborty, Rhyddhi, and Chhanda Chakraborti. 2015. *India, Health Inequities, and a Fair Health Care Provision: A Perspective from Health Capability* 16 (4): 567–580.

Coast, J., T. Flynn, L. Natarajan, K. Sproston, J. Lewis, Jordan J. Louviere, and Tim J. Peters. 2008. "Valuing the ICECAP Capability Index for Older People." *Social Science & Medicine* 67 (5): 874–882.

Diaz et al. 2015. An Analysis of the Intentions of a Chilean Disability Policy through the Lens of the Capability Approach. *Journal of Human Development and Capabilities* 16 (4): 483–500.

Feldman, Candace H., Gary L. Darmstadt, Vishwajeet Kumar, and Jennifer Prah Ruger. 2015. "Women's Political Participation and Health: A Health Capability Study in Rural India." *Journal of Health Politics, Policy and Law* 40 (1): 101–164.

Fleurbaey, M. 2007. "Social Choice and Just Institutions: New Perspectives." *Economics and Philosophy* 23 (1): 15–43.

Kinghorn, P. 2010. "Developing a Capability Approach to Measure and Value Quality of Life: An Application to Chronic Pain." PhD thesis. School of Medicine, Health Policy & Practice, University of East Anglia.

Kinghorn. 2015. "Exploring Different Interpretations of the Capability Approach in a Health Care Context: Where next?" *Journal of Human Development and Capabilities* 16 (4): 600–616.

Kuklys, W. 2005. *Amartya Sen's Capability Approach: Theoretical Insights and Empirical Applications*. Berlin: Springer Science & Business Media.

Lorgelly, P., et al. 2008. *The Capability Approach: Developing an Instrument for Evaluating Public Health Interventions*. University of Glasgow.

Mitra, S. 2006. "The Capability Approach and Disability." *Journal of Disability Policy Studies* 16 (4): 236–247.

Mitra, S. Forthcoming. "Measuring Disability and Wellbeing using the Capability Approach." In *Disability Social Rights*, edited by Stein, M.A., and M. Langford. Cambridge: Cambridge University Press.

Mitra, S., A. Posarac, and B. Vick. 2013. "Disability and Poverty in Developing Countries: A Multidimensional Study." *World Development* 41: 1–18.

Moczadlo. et al. 2015. "Corporate Contributions to Developing Health Capabilities." *Journal of Human Development and Capabilities* 16 (4): 549–566.

Mutanga, Oliver, and Melanie Walker. 2015. "Towards a Disability-Inclusive Higher Education Policy through the Capabilities Approach." *Journal of Human Development and Capabilities* 16 (4): 501–517.

Nguyen, Kim Thuy, Oanh Thi Hai Khuat, Shuangge Ma, Duc Cuong Pham, Giang Thi Hong Khuat, and Jennifer Prah Ruger. 2012a. "Effect of Health Expenses on Household Capabilities and Resource Allocation in a Rural Commune in Vietnam." *PLoS One* 7 (10): e47423.

Nguyen, Kim Thuy, Oanh Thi Hai Khuat, Shuangge Ma, Duc Cuong Pham, Giang Thi Hong Khuat, and Jennifer Prah Ruger. 2012b. "Impact of Health Insurance on Health Care Treatment and Cost in Vietnam: A Health Capability Approach to Financial Protection." *American Journal of Public Health* 102 (8): 1450–1461.

Nguyen, Kim Thuy, Oanh Thi Hai Khuat, Shuangge Ma, Duc Cuong Pham, Giang Thi Hong Khuat, and Jennifer Prah Ruger. 2012c. "Coping with Health Care Expenses Among Poor Households: Evidence from a Rural Commune in Vietnam." *Social Science & Medicine* 74 (5): 724–733.

Nussbaum, M. 2006. *Frontiers of Justice: Disability, Nationality, Species Membership*. Cambridge, MA: The Belknap Press of Harvard University Press.

Ruger, Jennifer Prah. 1998. "Aristotelian Justice and Health Policy: Capability and Incompletely Theorized Agreements." PhD diss., Harvard University.

Ruger, Jennifer Prah. 2004. "Health and Social Justice." *Lancet* 364 (9439): 1075–1080.

Ruger, Jennifer Prah. 2006. "Ethics and Governance of Global Health Inequalities." *Journal of Epidemiology and Community Health* 60 (11): 998–1002.

Ruger, Jennifer Prah. 2010. "Health Capability: Conceptualization and Operationalization." *American Journal of Public Health* 100 (1): 41–49.

Ruger, Jennifer Prah. 2015. "Health Economics and Ethics and the Health Capability Paradigm." *Journal of Human Development and Capabilities* 16 (4): 581–599.

Ruger, Jennifer Prah, and Kim Hak-Ju. 2006. "Global Health Inequalities: An International Comparison." *Journal of Epidemiology and Community Health* 60 (11): 928–936.

Sen, A. K. 1985. *Commodities and Capabilities, Professor Dr. P. Hennipman Lectures in Economics: Theory, Institutions, Policy, Volume 7*. Amsterdam: Elsevier.

Sen, A. K. 2009a. *The Idea of Justice*. Cambridge, MA: The Belknap Press of Harvard University Press.

Sen, A. K. 2009b. *Forward to Health and Social Justice*. Oxford: Oxford University Press.

Simon, J., P. Anand, et al. 2013. "Operationalising the Capability Approach for Outcome Measurement in Mental Health Research." *Social Science & Medicine*. Advance online publication. doi:10.1016/j.socscimed.2013.09.019.

Terzi, L. 2005. "Beyond the Dilemma of Difference: The Capability Approach on Disability and Special Educational Needs." *Journal of Philosophy of Education* 39 (3): 443–459.

Trani J. F., P. Bakshi, N. Bellanca, M. Biggeri, and F. Marchetta. 2011. "Disabilities through the Capability Approach Lens: Implications for Public Policies." *ALTER European Journal of Disability Research* 5 (3): 143–157.

Trani, Jean-Francois, Parul Bakhshi, Sarah Myers Tlapek, Dominique Lopez, and Fiona Gall. 2015. "Disability and Poverty in Morocco and Tunisia: A Multidimensional Approach." *Journal of Human Development and Capabilities* 16 (4): 518–548.

Trani, J. F., and T. Cannings. 2013. "Child Poverty in an Emergency and Conflict Context: A Multidimensional Profile and an Identification of the Poorest Children in Western Darfur?" *World Development* 48: 48–70.

An Analysis of the Intentions of a Chilean Disability Policy Through the Lens of the Capability Approach

ALVARO DÍAZ RUIZ, NATALIA SÁNCHEZ DURÁN & ALEXIS PALÁ

ABSTRACT *This article sheds light on the public policy situation for persons with severe disabilities in Chile by analyzing the Ministry of Health "Home-Based Care Program for Persons with Severe Disabilities." The article further advocates for the relevance of the Capability Approach (CA) in the assessment of public policy for persons with disabilities and intends to illustrate a link between a real policy and basic concepts of the CA providing a model of content analysis for public policy through the lens of the CA. We present a content analysis, focused on underlying intentions of agency, freedom, well-being, and achievement based in the official text of the Chilean program. Then we examine this content under original categories and matrices based on the work of Sen, to ultimately reveal how a current Chilean policy falls short of fully addressing the diagnosed situation of its target population and highlights areas for improvement. Not only does the program lack coherence and compliance with Chilean laws and international standards, but it also lacks connections with important concepts for persons in situations of dependency such as agency and freedom.*

1. Introduction

Disability is a multifaceted, complex concept. Internationally, the most widely accepted and recognized definition of disability for public policy is provided by the United Nations' Convention on the Rights of Persons with Disabilities (CRPD). The CRPD defines disability as an evolving concept that, "results from the interaction between persons with long-term physical, mental, intellectual or sensory impairments and the environmental barriers that hinder their full and effective participation in society" (UN 2007). This definition illustrates how a disability is often due to prejudice and the inaccessibility of an environment, instead of people's physical differences or medical issues (Ablon 2010).

This new perspective shifts away from attributing a disability solely to an individual, and recognizes how environments can disable. Globally, changes in public policy are critical in order to decrease the barriers to inclusion that persons with disabilities currently face and provide them with their rights to social protections (UN 2007, Art. 28). Poverty is all too often an obstacle for many people with disabilities. So much so that, Sen (2009) deems disability and poverty as inextricably linked. Out of the one billion people in the world estimated to be living with a disability, approximately 80% live in developing countries (WHO-World Bank 2011).

In 2004, the First National Survey of Disability (ENDISC)[1] conducted in Chile found that 12.9% of the population has some form of disability. The survey also revealed that 1 in 5 people who live in the lowest socioeconomic group of society has a disability (FONADIS 2006), while the rates are 1 in 8 for the middle group of society and 1 in 21 for the highest socioeconomic group of society (FONADIS-INE 2004).

Furthermore, the survey found that 2.5% of the Chilean population has a severe disability; that is, more than 400 000 people are "severely impaired and unable to function in their daily life without the care or support of a third party, and cannot manage to overcome their surrounding barriers alone, or do so with great difficulty," most of them living in the lowest socioeconomic group (FONADIS-INE 2004).

For the purposes of this article, our focus is on persons with severe disabilities (PWSD) in "situations of dependency," defined as "a specific type of disability in which two elements are present: a limitation of the individual to perform a specified activity, and the interaction of certain environmental factors related to personal and/or technical support," (Querejeta González 2004a, 27, 2004b, 349–350). It is also necessary to note that currently there is no existing data that relate type of disability to the respective situation of dependency besides the 2004 ENDISC (Díaz 2013).

The policy of the Ministry of Health (Ministerio de Salud, MINSAL) that is analyzed in this article is one of the few Chilean policies that target persons with disabilities in situations of dependency or bedridden. The purpose of this article is to utilize the Capability Approach (CA) to create a new model for the content analysis that permits an examination of a current Chilean public policy.

1.1. Public Policy and Dependency in Chile

The 2010 Chilean Law No. 20.422 (Ley No. 20.422 2010) derived from Chile's ratification of the CRPD in 2008 and established "Norms on Equal Opportunities and Social Inclusion of People with Disabilities," updating Chilean concepts of disability and inclusion to those established internationally and giving way to more active governmental engagement in terms of equal opportunities initiatives and more concrete actions for persons with disabilities.

Despite these advances, a great weakness remains in Chile's social protection system for adults (18–60 years old) with disabilities (Sánchez 2013). Public services in Chile mainly cover attention, care, and response for children and adolescents (0–24 years old)[2] or seniors (over 60 years old). This creates a significant void of support for adults with disabilities between the ages of 24 and 60 years. Even though a person with a disability could be living in a "situation of dependency," because of their age they are considered "independent" in the eyes of the law.

For this article, "independence" is the power to do something without the help of a third party and "personal autonomy" is a person's ability to self-govern, "administer or manage their dependency" (Querejeta Gonzalez 2004a, 36, 2004b, 353; Le Gall and Ruet 1996). Living in a situation of dependency may or may not result in the loss or diminution of personal autonomy. If a person living in a situation of dependency can administer and manage their dependency, they would preserve the power to decide what, how, and when to perform an action, which should be the ultimate goal. However, in Chile it is found that in situations of dependency, often autonomy is diminished (Díaz 2013).

1.2. Disability and the CA

Originally, Sen did not develop the CA to specifically address disability; rather disability was used to illustrate what the approach proposed (Mitra 2006).[3] However, many scholars of the CA have explored disability within this framework and find that "the capability approach has significant strengths in addressing disability issues," (Qizilbash 2006, 3) since it considers the multiple dimensions of a disability, such as the social and economic statuses of individuals. In *The Idea of Justice*, Sen himself states that, "the relevance of disability in the understanding of deprivation in the world is often underestimated, and this can be one of the most important arguments for paying attention to the capability perspective" (2009, 258).

While viewing disability through the lens of the CA, "the idea of equality is confronted by two kinds of diversity: (1) the basic heterogeneity of human beings, and (2) the multiplicity of variables in terms of which equality can be judged" (Sen 1992, 1). Deficiency of the body and/or the mind is only one among many variables that interact with a person's social, economic, and physical environment to produce a range of advantages or disadvantages, "disability is therefore a particular form of the general phenomenon of capability–poverty" (Burchardt 2004, 746).

Additionally, the CA takes into account the choices available to an individual. It emphasizes not only what a person is or does, their "functionings," but also the range of capabilities which they can choose from, that is the "set of capabilities" that a person can freely act upon. This perspective captures a person's relationship with their surrounding environment, as well as the available societal opportunities. Due to its comprehensiveness, the CA is believed to complement and exceed other disability models (Trani and Bakhshi 2009), which made it crucial to this analysis.

2. Fundamentals of Analysis

The analysis looked for conditions that created and/or enhanced a person's capabilities and their ability to act autonomously by searching for intentions of agency, freedom, well-being, and achievement present in the text of MINSAL's "Home-Based Care Program for Persons with Severe Disabilities." Ultimately, this analysis introduces a model for future content analyses of public policy through the lens of the CA. Due to the importance of freedom and agency[4] to the CA, we saw it as opportune and critical to select a government program aimed at addressing the needs of persons in situations of dependency since the ability to act autonomously, and the freedom to choose from a set of capabilities, is especially fragile for those living in situations of dependency.

In the Chilean context, an analysis of actions targeted at persons in situations of dependency acquires a special relevance due to the collectivist nature of society. Collectivism is a, "strong interdependence among members," where, "the interest of the group supersedes the interest of individuals, and becomes comprehensive to identity" (Marfull-Jensen and Flanagan 2014, 1). Collectivism in itself is not problematic, but becomes problematic in Chile because it creates a system heavily reliant on familial support and care for success. Furthermore, a collectivist mentality contrasts with the goals of autonomy and independence as outlined in the CRPD and Law No. 20.422, yet, as we will show, it continues to be reflected in public policies targeting persons with disabilities.

The following sections provide the various concepts that are critical for understanding and interpreting our analysis, results, and conclusions. It should be noted that the following analysis is far from a traditional analysis of public policy and constitutes an exploration within a methodology specifically crafted to analyze this type of social policy. Furthermore, the analysis was only performed on the official text of the selected relatively young program and cannot provide information on the program's implementation due to the absence of available data.

2.1. Basic Concepts

Utilizing the CA in public policy is not novel (Nussbaum 1997). The United Nations' Human Development Reports and the Sarkozy Commission are just a few examples of current policy initiatives that utilized the CA as a theoretical framework (Goerne 2010). For the purposes of this article, we assume that human flourishing is the end goal of any political activity, which means that the, "expan[sion] of freedom is both the primary end, and principal means of public policy: consequently, public policy should focus on removing barriers to freedom that leave people with little choice to exercise their reasoned agency" (Ruger 2009, 2).

According to Sen (1992), the achievement of equality should be evaluated in terms of the life that a person is capable of living. That is to say that equality should be measured by a person's freedom and agency—what they can actually say, be, and do in their lives. "Freedom is one of the most powerful social ideas and its relevance to the analysis of equality and justice is far reaching and strong" (96). More specifically, a close examination should be given to a person's rights, freedoms, and real opportunity. This is because equality "may be better represented by the freedom that the person has, and not by, or at least entirely by, what the person achieves—in well-being or in terms of agency—on the basis of that freedom" (Sen 1987a, 1987b, 47). Examples of this kind of examination are assessing whether a person can, "live longer, escape from avoidable causes of death, is well nourished, able to read, write, communicate and participate in science and literary tasks, etc." (Acosta 2011, 192). Arguably, "the creation of social opportunities makes a direct contribution to the expansion of human capabilities and quality of life" (Sen 1999, 144). The CA is a powerful tool that can help enhance citizens' lives through social opportunity, but "functionings and capabilities also need direct policy support" (Burchardt 2005, 369).

Typically within public policy, "equal opportunity" is understood as a person's disposition to a particular resource, barrier, or restriction. Within the CA, "equal opportunity" refers to the equality of capability, or the elimination of blatant inequality of capability, so that

> societal arrangements, involving many institutions (the state, the market, the legal system, political parties, the media, public interest groups and public discussion forums, among others) are investigated in terms of their contribution to enhancing and guaranteeing the substantive freedoms of individuals, seen as active agents of change, rather than as passive recipients of dispensed benefits. (Sen 1999, xii–xiii)

Sen (1993) indicates that it is possible to establish four points of interest when assessing human advantage, based on two different distinctions:

(1) First distinction:
  (a) The promotion of the person's well-being;
  (b) The search for the goals of the person's agency (what a person can say, be, and do), which may include goals other than the person's well-being.
(2) Second distinction:
  (a) Achievement, as in what a person actually reaches or performs;
  (b) Freedom or real opportunity to choose and achieve a valued goal.

When considering both distinctions together four concepts emerge: (1) "achievement of well-being," (2) "achievement of agency," (3) "freedom of wellbeing," and (4) "agency of freedom." Originally, Sen conceived of agency and well-being as distinct, but interconnected, aspects of the human life that command both respect and attention. As a result, agency and well-being have two dimensions: actual achievements and freedom of those achievements (Crocker 2006). To fulfill these dimensions,

> the ethically-sensitive analyst evaluates development policies and practices in the light of the extent to which they promote, protect, and restore human agency rather than merely the good or bad things that happen to people. (Crocker 2006, 298)

2.1.1. Well-being. Well-being can simply be defined as a person's achieved goals, but it more specifically pertains to evaluating a person's achievements in relation to their desired functionings. However, opportunities (functionings) are not weighted and valued solely by achieved goals (well-being); it is possible to have a real advantage and waste it, to sacrifice one's own well-being for the goals of another, or to not make use of the freedom to achieve a greater well-being (Sen 1987a, 1987b).

Well-being is of great importance to the analysis of social inequality and the assessment of public policy. Societies may accept the responsibility to help with their citizen's well-being, especially when there is some danger or vulnerability; for example, if someone is dying of hunger or cannot obtain adequate medical treatment. Providing a social service does not necessarily interfere with the citizen's other agency objectives (Sen 1992).

Within the context of public policy, well-being comprises the relevant functionings that every person, regardless of socioeconomic status, recognizes the worth of even if not prioritized by the individual (Burchardt 2005; Sen 1985). This is because, "problems of social injustice and inequity between different classes and groups relate strongly to extensive disparities in wellbeing—including the freedom that we respectively enjoy to achieve well-being" (Sen 1992, 72).

2.1.2. Agency. Agency refers to, "what a person is free to do and achieve in pursuit of whatever goal or values he or she regards as important" (Sen 1985, 203). Although agency is likely to overlap with and influence well-being, "since most people wish to promote their own well-being," (Burchardt 2005, 295) it is neither limited to well-being nor suggests a direct relationship between the two (Sen 1985). The "achievement of agency" is the successful completion of a person's valued goals and objectives, regardless of well-being (Sen 1992). This is because, at times, "[a]n expansion of freedom of agency can go with a reduction in actual well-being" (Sen 1985, 207). For example, someone can choose not to pursue their well-being, or engage in prejudicial actions towards their own well-being such as a person who drowns trying to save someone else's life (Burchardt 2005).

Moreover, attention needs to be given to the differences between agency and well-being in regard to freedom. "Freedom of agency" is, "one's freedom to bring about the achievements one values and which one attempts to produce" (Sen 1992, 57). Furthermore, it is the freedom to choose and achieve one's desires, free from external coercion or internal compulsion (Crocker 2006, 297). While "freedom of wellbeing" refers to "one's freedom to achieve those things that are constitutive of one's wellbeing" (Sen 1992, 57).

Finally, it is possible to distinguish between: (1) the "success of achieved agency," which is the occurrence of something that a person values independent of her role at the time of realization and (2) the "success of instrumental agency," which is the occurrence of such things by one's own effort, or where one has played an active role in its execution (Sen 1992, 56).

2.2. MINSAL: Home-Based Care Program for Persons with Severe Disability

There are only two policies in Chile directed at persons in situations of dependency: (1) SENADIS[5] "Promotion of the Autonomy and Attention to Dependency" and (2) MINSAL's "Home-Based Care Program for Persons with Severe Disabilities." With an estimated 2014 budget of 7500 million CLP[6] (12 million USD), MINSAL's program is the largest in terms of history, coverage, and financial resources, and for those reasons it was the policy selected for this analysis. Furthermore, SENADIS' policy is still in its piloting stages with a budget a tenth of the size of MINSAL's.

MINSAL established the Home-Based Care Program for Persons with Severe Disabilities in 2006 during President Michelle Bachelet's first term. The program provides detailed guidelines for the support of the elderly or other bedridden individuals as well as their caregivers. Moreover, the policy has two core components: one linked to in-home care services, and the other is more subsidiary, consisting of a monthly cash transfer of 22 000 CLP (40 USD), which is less than 10% of the average minimum wage salary in Chile (about 450 USD).

Overall, the intention of the program is, "to give the person with a severe disability, their caregivers, and family members, comprehensive in-home care in physical, emotional, and social ways that improve quality of life, thus enhancing recovery and/or autonomy" (MINSAL 2011, 5). At its simplest, this program is a health-care strategy or handbook implemented at the national level. Its success is highly dependent upon local administrations and health services utilizing their public health networks to extend coverage families and PWSD in situations of dependency. People with severe physical, mental or even multiple disabilities are especially vulnerable and in need of coverage since they frequently fall within the ranges of legal poverty (Sánchez 2013).

3. Methodology

The purpose for analyzing MINSAL's "Home-Based Care Program for Persons with Severe Disabilities" is to better understand the "underlying" (Bardin 1996, 104) Chilean interest in disability through the lens of the CA since the CA aligns with the program's goals of enhancing quality of life and personal autonomy. To do so, we performed a content analysis that searched for CA concepts and analyzed for intentions underlying the social practice and material surface of the text (Piñuel Raigada 2002). More specifically, our analysis looked for the presence of concepts and intentions related to the creation and/or enhancement of the capabilities of persons in situations of dependency, such as intentions of agency, freedom, well-being, and achievement (Holsti 1968). For this purpose, a series of matrices were developed with our categories and conceptual analysis.

A structural analysis was also performed. Units of diagnosis,[7] objectives, and components of the program were separated and analyzed in order to determine that our resulting categories were consistent, that is, if what was found in the structural analysis was also present in the objectives and components of our content analysis as well. Fundamentally, the unit of study in the analysis is a group of words, such as sentences or paragraphs, in the program that referenced the promotion, development, and/or strengthening of a person's capability (Bardin 1996).

The content analysis consisted of four initial steps: (1) the identification of a benefit, incentive, or action in the program, (2) evaluating its objectives, (3) breaking down its components, and (4) analyzing its indicators. These steps allowed us to assess internal consistency and identify underlying implications of program initiatives. Finally, we concluded whether each of the four steps promoted agency, well-being, freedom, and achievement. We made use of the Technical Standard (MINSAL 2006) as an auxiliary for interpretation of the text of the program when additional clarification was needed. No other texts were used to conduct the analysis.

Operationally the analysis used the following steps:

- Recognizing groupings in the text that referenced benefits, incentives, or actions that enhance capability. Only those groups of words that dealt directly with people with disabilities were considered and were distinguished in the text by expressions such as: "provide persons with disabilities," "the person with disabilities develop," "person's with a disability will receive" and other similar phrases. Additionally, we analyzed sets of words that referred to social structures, in terms of conversion factors that strived to create and enhance persons' capabilities (Goerne 2010).
- Semantically categorizing the data (Bardin 1996): related to agency, well-being, freedom, and achievement to decipher whether or not the program encourages the development of these concepts.

The analysis utilized simple matrices (Strauss and Corbin 2008) to consolidate our findings and separate the most important variables. The following divisions were established:

- Dimension: the identified goal of the Chilean state's action.
- Category: the type of services offered by the program to achieve said goal, taking into account how persons with disabilities receive them.
- Quotations: corresponds to actual phrasings that reveal the contents of the category in each stage of policy design (diagnosis, objectives, components, and indicators). Multiple phrasings can reference the same category.
- Elements of analysis: Are the theoretical contents of agency, well-being, freedom, and achievement there in the program? These are indicated by the mere presence, positive or negative, or absence of such content and were grouped as follows:
  - o Presence with positive effect (encourages its development): ✓
  - o Presence with negative effect (encourages that does not develop): X
  - o Absence (the item was not found): ø

4. Results

Our overall analysis revealed that MINSAL's policy has two principal goals or dimensions: in-home care for PWSD, and additional benefits that help provide more comprehensive care to PWSD. Furthermore, each dimension contains two distinct categories, or types of services, that we utilized to create our matrices (see Tables 1–4) for content analysis: "Direct Services Matrix," "Indirect Services Matrix," "Transfers Matrix," and "Networks Matrix". These four categories resulted from our assessment of all direct and indirect services with the objective of impacting the quality of life of PWSD, and were independently analyzed for intentions of: agency, well-being, freedom, and achievement. The detailed results of our analysis are broken down by matrix[8] category in the following subsections. Additionally, we use both "persons in situations of dependency" and "persons with severe disabilities" as interchangeable terms that reference the program's recipients or target population. Each matrix represents an action of MINSAL's program, which was analyzed by the intentions of: agency, well-being, freedom, and achievement.

4.1. Direct Services Matrix

The Direct Services Matrix (see Table 1) is part of the "in-home care for PWSD" policy dimension because it pertains to the services provided by the primary health teams in the homes of PWSD. These benefits are direct actions with economic costs (either in inputs, human resources, etc.) that exclusively target PWSD actions, but exclude direct transfers of cash.

The diagnosed problem of "direct services" is a need/demand for comprehensive care services for PWSD in Chile, which it attempts to address with the act of in-home care visits. However, in the text of MINSAL's policy there is a lack of explanation of what actions must be performed and why during those visits, instead these details are provided separately in the policy's Technical Standard (MINSAL 2006), making the actual text of the policy ambiguous and incomplete. The Technical Standard additionally provides a clearer definition of program's recipients, stating its target population as PWSD who "suffer" from severe dependence and require support, guidance and supervision in all daily activities, such as bathing, dressing, going to the bathroom, relocating, and eating. Additionally, the Technical Standard is the first direct reference to persons who are bedridden (MINSAL 2006, 8). During the in-home care visits, health officials are supposed to comply with specified procedures, diagnose, and intervene based on mobility/disability of PWSD, aid with their daily activities, and conduct training sessions with caregivers to enhance awareness and knowledge.

Overall, direct services focus on the support of PWSD in situations of dependency. That support does lead to some achievement of well-being for the individual since the program helps the person to complete various personal needs, such as bathing, dressing, going to the bathroom, relocating, feeding, etc., but these personal needs represent the scope of well-being targeted.

Underlying the Technical Standard, we found an intention of freedom, since persons in situations of dependency can utilize the services provided to enhance their capability sets and access previously unattainable capabilities. It is important to note that the actual presence of freedom is contingent upon the recipient valuing those new capabilities. The content analysis found, that it was not possible to determine if in fact the associated capabilities were prioritized by the recipients.

Ultimately, the analysis found no intentions of agency associated with direct services. Rather, it can be argued that the individual's agency is violated since the objectives listed in the text of the program are to "take care" and "provide" for said person, and furthermore "intervene" and "transmit", as stated in the Technical Standard. Both documents define the health team as the central actors and the person in a situation of dependency as acted upon. There are no references to recipient's personal goals or if the newly attainable capabilities are those that the person values.

Even though the need for comprehensive care and services is stated in the original diagnosis for direct services, the text of the program never provides evidence to support these assertions and the established procedures of in-home care visits, such as research on what

Table 1. Direct Services Matrix.

Dimension	In-home care for PWSD			
Category: Direct services	Benefits that are directly aimed at PWSD. These services involve direct actions with economic costs (either in inputs, human resources, etc.), but are not direct transfers of cash			
	Diagnosis	Objectives	Components	Indicators
Process of analysis	"Must provide comprehensive services to individuals (and families), and even more so in segments of greater economic and social vulnerability" "The importance of primary care health teams … who must provide care for people who have some degree of disability" "They must provide services according to their needs" "This segment demand services and therefore, the existence of devices in their network to respond to those needs" "75.7% (of the population) receive attention and demand services in the public sector"	"Provide comprehensive care for people who have severe disabilities, considering the psychosocial needs of the patient and his family"	Provide homecare to address health needs of the PWSD Address health care holistically and look at biological as well as psychological needs of the PWSD and their family	1. Number of PWSD served organized by sex and age 2. Number of visits per-patient in comparison to number of scheduled visits 3. Percentage of patients with bedsores
Intentions of agency	X	X	X	X
Intentions of well-being	✓	✓	✓	✓
Intentions of freedom	ø	ø	ø	ø
Intentions of achievement	✓	✓	✓	✓
Internal coherence	• The program indicates the importance of providing care to all people with a disability. However, this program is exclusively for PWSD in situations of dependency who are bedridden since an indicator of quality of service is the percentage of patients with bedsores. • Emphasis is placed on "comprehensive care" and "quality of life" for persons with disabilities, but indicators only reveal coverage, which does not measure quality of care or even what types of services were provided.			

specific supports PWSD in Chile lack. The absence of evidence for direct services coupled with the lack of consideration of the recipient's agency led to weak objectives, and subsequently indicators that cannot definitively determine if the program's goals of autonomy and quality of life enhancement are achieved.

4.2. Indirect Services Matrix

The Indirect Services Matrix (see Table 2) is part of the "in-home care for PWSD" dimension because it pertains to the services provided by the primary health teams in the homes of PWSD, but these actions or benefits target caregivers or those related to PWSD. Like direct services, indirect services involve actions with economic cost (in inputs, human resources, etc.), but are not direct transfers of cash.

The analysis found that "indirect services" primarily refer to the achievement of well-being as well but actions categorized in this matrix target the well-being of the family or caregivers, thus indirectly affect the care recipient. The objective of this training is to provide caregivers with necessary tools to facilitate their work and overcome environmental challenges (MINSAL 2006, 7). This component of the program strives to improve the family's quality of life as well as the quality of care provided, since families are typically the main providers of care in Chile. Freedom is weakly present in the training's objectives since caregivers could further develop their capabilities to provide quality care to PWSD, but again, the analysis found no intentions of agency.

First, it is unclear whether the training is actually desired by the family members, and second whether the preferences and goals of the family members' align with those of the training program. Additionally, the program proclaims that it is based on the "shared responsibility of the family group," which implies that familial care ultimately is an obligation rather than a choice. Furthermore, PWSD do not qualify for the program without familial care, making the family's participation mandatory, which is problematic for more reasons than just agency. In the program's objectives, this obligation is downplayed; it is presented mildly as a combined strategy. However, it is very significant because without a family, a PWSD does not qualify for the program's support.

4.3. Transfers Matrix

The Transfers Matrix (see Table 3) is classified in the "additional benefits that help to provide more comprehensive care for PWSD" dimension. This dimension includes benefits that are not overt acts of care, and are not confined to the homes of PWSD. Furthermore, these are economic benefits that qualifying PWSD receive indirectly by the direct transfer of cash to caregivers.

The analysis found intentions of well-being present in the "Transfers Matrix." The program diagnosed the need for monetary support based on the statistic that one in five persons with a disability in Chile lives in the lowest socioeconomic sector of society. Again, this action is an indirect benefit to persons in a situation of dependency since the monetary payment is directly given to the caregivers. The primary goal of this monetary transfer is to help foster the well-being of the caregivers. This enhancement of financial resources is weakly freedom in the sense that it can permit the family to develop other capabilities that were previously inaccessible due to their need to work, but the monetary amount is meager and not supported in the text by evidence Additionally, it could allow the caregiver to, "exert greater control over the who, how and when of the assistance they need" Burchardt (2005, 748), but this support does not necessarily yield the achievement of any given functioning.

Table 2. Indirect Services Matrix.

Dimension	In-home care for PWSD			
Category: Indirect services	Actions or benefits aimed at caregivers or those related to PWSD. These indirect services involve an action with economic cost (either in inputs, human resources, etc.), but are not direct transfers of cash			
	Diagnosis	Objectives	Components	Indicators
Process of analysis	"Must provide comprehensive services to individuals (and families), and even more so in segments of greater economic and social vulnerability" "It is based on the shared responsibility that the family must assume in the care and attention of people with disabilities, because of this, the health team must deliver necessary tools to families, for the care of patients, and to engage the family in this process"	"Prepare the families who care for such patients, delivering holistic service with emphasis on the person, his family and their environment" "Give caregivers and families the necessary tools to provide comprehensive care for persons with severe disabilities"	Provide necessary tools and training to families and the PWSD surrounding environment	1. Trained and paid caregivers (number of trained caregivers who receive payment / total number of caregivers who receive payment)
Intentions of agency	X	X	ø	X
Intentions of well-being	✓	✓	ø	✓
Intentions of freedom	ø	✓	ø	ø
Intentions of achievement	✓	✓	ø	X
Internal coherence	• While there is coherence between the diagnosis and its objectives, there is a lack of consistency between components and indicators. The single component we have listed is, "provide necessary tools and training," but the measurement of that is payment to caregivers, which does accurately measure the goal of learning techniques or actions that increase the quality of life of the person. • This payment refers to the monetary benefits, which is not necessarily a tool and does not develop the skills or competencies of the caregivers that will improve the well-being of the PWSD.			

Table 3. Transfers Matrix.

Dimension Category:	Additional benefits that help provide more comprehensive care to PWSD[9]			
Money transfers	Indirect economic benefits for qualifying PWSD via their caregiver(s)			
	Diagnosis	Objectives	Components	Indicators
Process of analysis	"The study points out that for people living with a disability in Chile one of every five live in low socioeconomic status; one in eight people live in the middle socioeconomic status, and one person with a disability out of every 21 are of high socioeconomic status"	"To recognize the work of the caregivers of persons with severe disabilities, and provide training and monetary support if they fulfill the qualifying criteria"	Monetary support to the care providers of PWSD especially those in the range of poverty Recognize the work of these care providers by a set annual payment To receive payment, the recipient must be enrolled in their government health center, be a beneficiary of FONASA or of any government program, be classed as poor, destitute or not indigent through a social assessment by a social worker or application of tab CAS II team by the Social Assistance of the municipality.	1. Trained and paid caregivers (number of trained caregivers who receive payment / total number of caregivers who receive payment)
Intentions of agency	ø	ø	X	ø
Intentions of well-being	✓	✓	✓	✓
Intentions of freedom	ø	✓	✓	ø
Intentions of achievement	ø	ø	ø	ø
Internal coherence	• The text assumes that caregivers are part of the family and live in house or nearby. It also assumes that the socioeconomic conditions families are similar to those who care for the PWSD. • This monetary support is more like a reward for 'good behavior' or participation, which does not necessarily result in better care for the PWSD, or increase their capabilities since it is a set amount of money and not assessed by the varying situations and needs of PWSD. • The indicator is not clear about what exactly is measured. It illustrates how many caregivers receive payment but not the quality of life or effective capacity building that result from this payment.			

While the intent of well-being is evident throughout the various elements of the analysis, the intention of freedom is not as apparent in the program's diagnosis or indicators. Moreover, intentions of agency are missing from this action of the program and are arguably jeopardized. For example, the support could arguably incentivize social immobility since caregivers must maintain an indigent living situation in order to continue qualifying for monetary support.

4.4. Networks Matrix

The Networks Matrix (see Table 4) is included in the "additional benefits that help to provide more comprehensive care for PWSD" dimension since these benefits are not overt acts of care, and are not confined to the home of PWSD. Specifically, this matrix refers to direct or indirect societal benefit(s) for PWSD that result from the effective coordination between the government, private sector, agencies, families, and PWSD.

This category refers mainly to the achievement of well-being for persons in situations of dependency and their families. The emphasis placed on networks of (public, private, and social) support strives to improve quality of life, opportunity, and the continuation of health care for persons in situations of dependency. There is an achievement of well-being in regard to the concentration on the health of PWSD. However, the lack of coherence between the objectives stated in the diagnosis and its indicators does not allow the achievement of well-being to develop fully.

The analysis revealed a slight development of agency detailed in these program objectives, since the recipients have the opportunity to change health programs if they need to do so. Since this could be a desired goal of the person in a situation of dependency, it makes it an opportunity for agency exertion. However, it is important to emphasize that health care itself is not a final goal, but rather a means to obtain a goal or capability like health (Sen 1992, 36), so this does not ensure an enhancement in overall quality of life. Finally, there were no present indicators for the development of freedom, which would promote the development of capabilities or real opportunities.

5. Overall Findings

Ultimately, the content analysis concluded that the MINSAL program lacks coherence and does not ensure solutions to the problems of dependency it proclaims to address in its initial diagnosis. The program's declared intention is, "to give the person with a severe disability, their caregivers, and family members, comprehensive care at home in physical, emotional, and social ways aimed at improving quality of life, thus enhancing recovery and/or autonomy" (MINSAL 2011, 5). These shortcomings are to the detriment of the well-being, agency, freedom, and achievement of PWSD in situations of dependency.

5.1. Lack of Internal Consistency

The content analysis revealed a serious deficiency in the soundness of the MINSAL program. The text loses coherence between its components, so much so that the problem identified in the diagnosis is not fully addressed in by components or measured by indicators. Due to this, the program's objectives and components have the intentions to resolve targeted issues, but do not necessarily guarantee that the problem will be tackled. Additionally, the indicators do not take into account all the actions of the program's components, which prevents an evaluator from effectively assessing the program's impact. For example, an indicator of success for in-home care is a reduction in the percentage of PWSD

Table 4. Networks Matrix.

Dimension Category: Networks	Additional benefits that help provide more comprehensive care to PWSD. Perceived direct or indirect societal benefit(s) for PWSD that result from the effective coordination between the government, private sector, agencies, families, and PWSD			
	Diagnosis	Objectives	Components	Indicators
Process of analysis	"This segment demand services and therefore, the existence of devices in their network to respond to their needs" "It is essential to integrate the work of institutions dealing with the issue of disability, since they must provide critical services to individuals and families, even more so in sectors of greater economic and social vulnerability" "The development of networking strategies is essential, by which, ministries, services, and municipalities, as the civil society, must plan activities that aim to improve the quality of life of the person with disabilities and their families'" "75.7% (of the population) receive attention and demand services in the public sector"	"Safeguard the continuity and timeliness of a health-care network, making appropriate arrangements in the event that these services are needed" "Maintain updated database of persons with severe disabilities on a web page"	Each health facility must inform the Secretary of Care in the Ministry of Health, about implementing a program Follow the process of registry on the webpage and enter their Record Monthly Statistical REM	Updated Record in web page (No of Quotas used by the Health Service, registered in the web worksheet, estimated to complete year/No. of quotas committed by the Health Service)
Intentions of agency	ø	✓—ø	ø	X
Intentions of well-being	✓	✓	ø	X
Intentions of freedom	ø	ø	ø	X
Intentions of achievement	✓	✓	ø	X
Internal coherence	• There is a consensus across categories to address the need for integrated networks of services for PWSD, but it lacks an indicator. • There are specific activities listed in the text (p. 10), indicating that the health-care team should incorporate community resources such as volunteers, monitors, NGOs, or others, to create a larger network that can help perform follow-up efforts, develop care plans, and monitor records. • Although the maintenance of records is necessary in order to provide adequate services, it is an administrative action that does not necessarily provide a benefit to the PWSD, their caregivers, or improve their quality of life.			

with bedsores, but this indicator has neither a meaning for non-bedridden PWSD nor ensures the enhancement of quality of life and autonomy

5.2. Categories of Analysis Concerning the CA

The analysis discovered that intentions of freedom and agency are virtually absent and that there is at present a bias towards achievement and well-being. The program's components target caregivers instead of persons in situations of dependency, who are supposed to be the program's beneficiaries. Ultimately, persons in situations of dependency primarily indirectly benefit from the program, and their caregivers are those who truly receive direct benefits. This attests to the collectivist nature of Chilean society and its continual presence in policies despite contradiction to the CRPD and Law No. 20.422.

Furthermore, our analysis concluded that the program is fundamentally collectivistic (Marfull-Jensen and Flanagan 2014) since it attributes the role of primary caregivers to the family. The program was written in such a way that persons in situations of dependency and their caregivers are conceived as a single unit. Primarily families, rather than persons in situations of dependency, are the direct actors and beneficiaries of the program; two integral components of the MINSAL policy, training and the stipend, are exclusively offered to families. In the context of this policy, the collectivist mentality assumes that the benefit to one would be of benefit to the other; this occurrence cannot easily be controlled, especially since our analysis found weak, incoherent indicators, and virtually no oversight due to the absence of established follow-up mediations to ensure continuous benefit for persons in situations of dependency. As a result, the infiltration of collectivism and lack of coherence between the program's diagnoses, components, and indicators, discard the agency, autonomy, and functionings of persons in situations of dependency and ultimately impair the program from assuring the enhancement of the autonomy and quality of life for persons in situations of dependency.

Ultimately, the program does not deliver solutions to the problems of dependency it proclaims to address in its initial diagnosis. The program's declared intention is, "to give the person with a severe disability, their caregivers, and family members, comprehensive care at home in physical, emotional, and social ways aimed at improving quality of life, thus enhancing recovery and/or autonomy" (MINSAL 2011, 5). Truly, as we have shown, the family/caregivers are the direct beneficiaries of this program, and the agency, autonomy, and functionings of the person in a situation of dependency are not considered.

6. Discussion

Currently, disability is not integrated into the Chilean social protection system. Instead, there are various social services available to persons with disabilities, such as pensions, forms of technical assistance, and other monetary supports. Even it was not until MINSAL's Home-Based Care Program for Persons with Severe Disabilities in 2006 that the Chilean government recognized and attempted to provide support to persons in situations of dependency. Even though the MINSAL's program is a relatively new policy, a content analysis of this program suggests that it fails to fully address the diagnosed situation. In order to truly achieve its goal of enhancing the autonomy and well-being of persons in situations of dependency, the policy requires redesign, scheduled implementation, and furthermore, the political will to position this issue on the policy agenda and advance it in the realm of social protection.

Overall, in order to foster well-being and promote the autonomy of this population, a reform of public policy is critical and necessary within the framework and understanding of the CA. The well-being of persons in situations of dependency, and even the current success of the MINSAL's policy, rests problematically upon families and diminishes the autonomy of its target population in various ways. Although it provides some necessary supports that may enhance persons' capability sets, such as assistance with bathroom and mobility, it is uncertain whether these supports actually increase well-being, and the indicators fail to measure impact as well. Unintentionally, this renders the policy vulnerable to maintaining persons in situations of dependency in disabling environments where capabilities and functionings are impaired (Burchardt 2004; Mitra 2006). The valued functionings of persons in situations of dependency are not considered, which prevents persons from exercising their agency, becoming more autonomous, and even assessing the state of their personal well-being. In order to more securely achieve the enhancement of well-being and autonomy for persons with disabilities, future policies must give special attention to the concepts of agency and freedom, which are virtually absent from MINSAL's policy. Due to its collectivist influences MINSAL's policy lacked agreement with both national and international laws.

The challenge seems to lie in the lack of political and technical awareness of these established laws and the need to develop policies that promote the personal autonomy and agency of persons in situations of dependency. Visions of assistance and charity permeate the language and practice of public policy for this population, which further goes against what is promoted in Law No. 20.422 and the CRPD. Furthermore, it seems important to teach policy-makers to view persons with disabilities, whether mild or severe, as autonomous, valid subjects in the decision-making process in order to guarantee their agency and self-determination with choices that affect their quality of life and well-being.

Additionally, consideration needs to be given to the freedom of persons in situations of dependency in order to ensure respect of the actions that recipients' value, and to diminish the decision-making power that caregivers currently possess. Even though freedom, autonomy, and agency can appear problematic within the context of people who are to some degree dependent upon their caregivers, it is achievable and needs to be protected and promoted by policy (Burchardt 2005). The necessity of this redesign is made apparent when adults with disability and dependency "find themselves in a situation of exception to their originally projected lifecycle [… and], the protection and assurance of those individuals rests essentially on the family" (Sánchez 2013, 95). What happens when there is no family, either because of abandonment, or because the individual has outlived them? These "exceptions" are excluded from the support of the MINSAL's policy, but most likely are in dire need.

Disclosure statement

No potential conflict of interest was reported by the authors.

Notes

1. At the time this article was written this was the most current national data.
2. People with disabilities in Chile can remain in the school system until the age of 24.
3. For examples see: Sen (1987a, 1987b, 1992, 1999, 2004a, 2004b, 2004c, 2004d, 2009) and Nussbaum (2000, 2003, 2006, 2011).
4. Additionally, the two programs selected are the only ones dedicated to adults with disabilities, regardless of age group.
5. *Servicio Nacional de la Discapacidad*, National Service for Disability.
6. Chilean Pesos.
7. Diagnosis in public policy analysis must be understood as the way to identify elements and relationships for analysis (Sabatier 2007; Dunn 2008).

8. With the matrices, the reader must consider the description of elements provided in the last paragraph of the previous section.
9. Unlike the dimension of services, public benefits are passive in that they do not represent overt actions of care for people with disabilities; examples are tax rebates on certain goods, preferential access to subsidies, transfers, pensions, bonds, etc.

References

Ablon, Joan. 2010. *Brittle Bones, Stout Hearts and Minds: Adults with Osteogenesis Imperfecta*. Sudbury, MA: Jones and Bartlett Print.

Acosta, Alberto. 2011. "Sólo Imaginando Otros Mundos, Se Cambiará Éste: Reflexiones sobre el Buen Vivir." In *Vivir Bien: ¿Paradigma No Capitalista?*, edited by H. Farah and L. Vasapollo, 189–208. La Paz: Plural Editores.

Bardin, Laurence. 1996. *Análisis de Contenido* (C. Suárez, Trad.). Madrid: Ediciones Akal.

Burchardt, Tania. 2004. "Capabilities and Disability: The Capabilities Framework and the Social Model of Disability." *Disability & Society* 19 (7): 735–751. doi:10.1080/0968759042000284213.

Burchardt, Tania. 2005. *Incomes, Functionings and Capabilities: The Well-Being of Disabled People in Britain*. London: London School of Economics.

Crocker, David. 2006. "Sen and Deliberative Democracy." In *Capabilities Equality: Basic Issues and Problem*, edited by Alexander Kaufman, 155–97. New York: Routlege.

Díaz, Álvaro. 2013. "Elementos para una Política de Dependencia en Chile." In *Políticas Públicas para la Dependencia*, edited by SENADIS, Álvaro Díaz Ruiz, and Natalia Sánchez, 23–35. Santiago: Servicio Nacional de la Dicapacidad.

Dunn, William. 2008. *Public Policy Analysis: An Introduction*. Upper Saddle River, NJ: Pearson Prentice Hall.

FONADIS. 2006. *Discapacidad en Chile: Pasos Hacia Un Modelo Integral del Funcionamiento Humano*. Santiago, Chile: Gobierno de Chile, Fondo Nacional de la Discapacidad. www.senadis.gob.cl/descarga/i/633/documento

FONADIS-INE. 2004. *Primer Estudio Nacional de la Discapacidad en Chile ENDISC*. Santiago, Chile: Fondo Nacional de la Discapacidad (FONADIS) e Instituto Nacional de Estadísticas (INE). http://www.ine.cl/canales/chile_estadistico/encuestas_discapacidad/pdf/presentacion.pdf.

Goerne, Alexander. 2010. *The Capability Approach in Social Policy Analysis: Yet Another Concept? European Comission, Dissemination and Dialogue Centre*. Edinburgh: RECWOWE Publication.

Holsti, Ole Rudolf. 1968. "Content Analysis." In *The Handbook of Social Psychology*, edited by G. Lindzey and E. Aronson, 596–692. Reading: Addison-Wesley.

Le Gall, Michel, and Jean-Louis, Ruet. 1996. "Evaluación y análisis de la autonomía." *Enciclopedia Médico-Quirúrgica, 26-030-A-10* .

Ley No. 20.422. 2010. *Establece Normas sobre Igualdad de Oportunidades e Inclusión Social de Personas con Discapacidad*. Santiago, Chile: Ministerio de Planificación. http://bcn.cl/1m09d.

Marfull-Jensen, Marisol, and Tara Flanagan. 2014. "The 2010 Chilean National Disability Law: Self-Determination in a Collectivistic Society." *Journal of Disability Policy Studies* 1 (9). doi: 10.1177/1044207314533384.

MINSAL. 2006. *Norma de Cuidados Domiciliarios de Personas que Sufren de Discapacidad Severa*. Santiago, Chile: Ministerio de Salud. https://www.ssmaule.cl/paginas/index.php?option=com_docman&task=doc_download&gid=2154&Itemid=123.

MINSAL. 2011. *Programa de Atención Domiciliaria a Personas con Discapacidad Severa* (Resolucion Exenta 91/2011). Santiago, Chile: Ministerio de Salud, Subsecretaria de Redes Asistenciales. https://cesfamsi.files.wordpress.com/2011/04/programa-atencic3b3n-domiciliaria-2011.doc.

Mitra, Sophie. 2006. "The Capability Approach and Disability." *Journal of Disability Policy Studies* 16 (4): 236–247.

Nussbaum, Martha. 1997. "Capabilities and Human Rights." *Fordham Law Review* 66 (2): 273–300.

Nussbaum, Martha. 2000. *Women and Women Development: The Capabilities Approach*. Cambridge: Cambridge University Press.

Nussbaum, Martha. 2003. "Capabilities as Fundamental Entitlements: Sen and Social Justice." *Feminist Economics* 9 (2–3): 33–59.

Nussbaum, Martha. 2006. *Frontiers of Justice: Disability, Nationality, Species Membership*. Cambridge, Massachusetts: Harvard University Press.

Nussbaum, Martha. 2011. *Creating Capabilities: The Human Development Approach*. Cambridge, MA: Harvard University Press.

Piñuel Raigada, José Luis. 2002. "Epistemología, Metodología y Técnicas del Análisis de Contenido." *Estudios de Sociolingüística* 3 (1): 1–42.

Qizilbash, Mozaffar. 2006. "Disability and Human Development." Paper prepared for the 2006 International HDCA Conference, Groningen, August 29–September 1.

Querejeta González, Miguel. 2004a. *Discapacidad/Dependencia. Unificación de Criterios de Valoración y Clasificación*. Madrid: Instituto de Migraciones y Servicios Sociales IMSERSO. http://sid.usal.es/idocs/F8/FDO7174/Discapacidad_dependencia.pdf.

Querejeta González, Miguel. 2004b. "Aportaciones de la CIF a la Conceptualización de la Dependencia." *Rehabilitación* 38 (6): 348–354.

Ruger, Jennifer Prah. 2009. *Health and Social Justice*. Kindle ed. Oxford: Oxford University Press.

Sabatier, Paul. 2007. *Theories of the Policy Process*. Boulder, CO: Westview Press.

Sánchez, Natalia. 2013. "Corresponsabilidad público-privada en el cuidado de personas con discapacidad mental en situación de dependencia en Chile." M.A Thesis, Universidad de Chile. http://tesis.uchile.cl/handle/2250/115484.

Sen, Amartya. 1985. "Well-Being, Agency and Freedom: The Dewey Lectures 1984." *The Journal of Philosophy* 82 (4): 169–221

Sen, Amartya. 1987a. *Commodities and Capabilities*. 19th ed. New Delhi: Oxford University Press.

Sen, Amartya. 1987b. *On Ethics and Economics*. New Delhi: Oxford University Press.

Sen, Amartya. 1992. *Inequality Reexamined*. Cambridge, MA: Harvard University Press.

Sen, Amartya. 1993. "Capability and Well Being." In *The Quality of Life*, edited by M. Nussbaum and A. Sen, 30–53. Oxford: Clarendon Press.

Sen, Amartya. 1999. *Development as Freedom*. New York: Anchor Books.

Sen, Amartya. 2004a. "Disability and Justice." Keynote Speech presented at the conference Disability and Inclusive Development: Sharing, Learning and Building Alliances, organized by the World Bank, Washington, November 30–December 1, 2004.

Sen, Amartya. 2004b. "Elements of a Theory of Human Rights." *Philosophy and Public Affairs* 32 (4): 315–356.

Sen, Amartya. 2004c. "Why Health Equity." In *Public Health, Ethics, and Equity*, edited by S. Anand, F. Peter, and A. Sen, 21–33. Oxford: Oxford University Press.

Sen, Amartya. 2004d. "Health Achievement and Equity: External and Internal Perspectives." In *Public Health, Ethics, and Equity*, edited by S. Anand, F. Peter, and A. Sen, 263–278. Oxford: Oxford University Press.

Sen, Amartya. 2009. *The Idea of Justice*. Cambridge, MA: Belknap of Harvard UP.

Strauss, Anaselm, and Juliet Corbin. 2008. *Basics of Qualitative Research: Grounded Theory Procedures and Techniques*. California, CA: SAGE Publications, Inc.

Trani, Jean F., and Parul Bakhshi. 2009. "Lack of a Will or of a Way? Taking a Capability Approach for Analysing Disability Policy Shortcomings and Ensuring Programme Impact in Afghanistan." Working Paper Series: No. 10. Leonard Cheshire Disability and Inclusive Development Centre, UCL. https://www.ucl.ac.uk/lc-ccr/centrepublications/workingpapers/WP10_Lack_of_a_will_or_of_a_way.pdf.

UN. 2007. Convention on the Rights of Persons with Disabilities: resolution/adopted by the General Assembly of the United Nations. http://www.refworld.org/docid/45f973632.html.

WHO-World Bank. 2011. *World Report on Disability*. Geneva: World Health Organization. http://www.who.int/disabilities/world_report/2011/report.pdf.

Towards a Disability-inclusive Higher Education Policy through the Capabilities Approach

OLIVER MUTANGA & MELANIE WALKER

ABSTRACT *Evidence from international literature shows that despite interventions and policies, students with disabilities face persistent challenges in higher education. The capabilities approach can take us forward in addressing these challenges in two ways. Nussbaum's version of the capabilities approach, in particular, provides us with an analytical framework to explore valued opportunities and freedoms from a social justice perspective. Secondly, in line with Sen's argument, the approach can serve as the informational base for disability policies. In this study, the capabilities approach is operationalized within education by applying Walker's list of eight valued freedoms and opportunities to students with disabilities. Data are drawn from a qualitative study examining the processes through which students with disabilities at two South African universities make their educational choices and negotiate different structures on their way to, and in higher education. These students identified key valued freedoms and opportunities that are needed to access and succeed in higher education. Four of the eight valued freedoms and opportunities on Walker's list emerged strongly in this study. Seven other valued freedoms and opportunities which fall outside of Walker's list were also identified. These 11 key valued freedoms and opportunities, we argue, are needed for the formulation of socially just disability-inclusive policies.*

Introduction

International studies on disability and higher education have shown that students with disabilities face significant challenges in higher education beyond those experienced by students without disabilities (Vickerman and Blundell 2010). Scholars point to a number of issues, including the role of social arrangements in perpetuating inequalities (Barnes and Mercer 2003; Oliver 1996), the effect of impairment on disability (Bury 2000; Shakespeare 2014) and the interplay between impairment and socio-economic arrangements in the lives of people with disabilities (Mitra 2014; Terzi 2005; Warnock, Norwich, and Terzi 2010). However, little is known about the specific experiences of students with disabilities in South African higher education (SAHE), given that the field is under-researched with only a small number of studies to provide the much needed data (DHET 2013). Nor do we have studies from a capabilities perspective. Thus far, most work on the lives of students with disabilities in higher education has viewed disability from the social model perspective. In an effort to distance themselves from the medical perspective or to discredit it, proponents of the social model have, in our view, neglected the need to understand people with disabilities' challenges not only emanating from the social environment but from other factors such as the individual, economic and political spheres. As a consequence of the limitations of existing perspectives to understanding disability, researchers' attention has now shifted to developing a better understanding of the multiple and intersecting social, political and cultural barriers which place obstacles in the way of access and success of students with disabilities in higher education (Fuller and Healey 2009; Strnadova, Hájková, and Květoňová 2015). Nonetheless, these studies do not extend to addressing the freedoms and opportunities that individual students with disabilities value in higher education. This is where we situate this paper using the capabilities approach as a frame of analysis to introduce a language of well-being and agency, while still taking account of the relationship between individual opportunities and social arrangements which shape students' ability to convert their means to achieve into freedoms and actual achievements.

The paper builds upon earlier studies that have analysed the lives of people with disabilities using the capabilities approach, although these have not been located in higher education. Most of these studies have either theorized disability issues (Mitra 2014; Terzi, 2005) or in the case of empirical studies, have utilized quantitative approaches (Mitra, Posarac, and Vick 2013; Trani et al. 2011; Trani and Canning 2013). This paper integrates theory and qualitative data and also adds to the literature on capabilities lists (Nussbaum 2011; Unterhalter 2003; Walker 2006; Wilson-Strydom 2015). The contributions of the capabilities approach to human development has been stated by many scholars, including Alkire (2008), who identifies two aspects, the normative role and the policy role. The normative role is concerned with which and whose capabilities are being expanded or hindered, while the policy role focuses on how and why capabilities either expand or are thwarted. However, policy-makers and practitioners are discouraged by the operational difficulties when it comes to applying the capabilities approach. We therefore show how capabilities could be operationalized in both higher education and the disability field, and because different information leads to different kinds of policies, why capabilities are important in providing the informational basis for social justice claims in disability research and practice. The paper seeks to answer a question that is yet to gain currency in both higher education and disability studies: what are the conditions and opportunities necessary for securing what students with disabilities value in higher education? This is timely because inequality is increasingly a source of public concern. Moreover, the sustainable development goals (SDGs) debate provides an opportunity to ground disability and education matters in a wider social justice agenda.

In the paper we firstly explore major issues discussed in recent studies on disability in higher education, both internationally and nationally. A discussion on the capabilities approach and how it has been used to frame disability follows. The third section gives context and the methodology of this study while the bulk of the paper presents and discusses the findings of the study.

Capabilities Approach, Disability and the Dilemma of Difference

The capabilities approach has been used to study many disability-related issues. Sen has been concerned with the economic well-being of persons with disabilities and mentions it repeatedly in his writings on the capabilities approach. Mobility equipment or other forms of resources and help required by people with disabilities may soak up a large proportion of income that would otherwise be adequate for both people without disabilities and those with disabilities (Sen 2009). He further outlines two disadvantages from which people with disabilities might suffer. He says that some people with disabilities have a *conversion handicap* that is, the difficulties in converting their resources or incomes into "good living" because of disability (Sen 2009, 258). Additionally, people with disabilities might suffer an *earning handicap* as they might need more income to achieve similar functionings as others, for example, to buy a wheelchair in order to be mobile. Other than Sen, the capabilities approach has been used by many scholars on disability-related issues other than economic well-being. A growing number of scholars (Mitra 2006; Nussbaum 2006; Reindal 2009; Terzi 2010) have used the capabilities approach to define disability. Within the capabilities perspective, brief, disability occurs when an individual with impairment is deprived of opportunities and freedoms to do what he or she values to do (Mitra 2006). Nussbaum (2006) argues that justice for people with disabilities should include whatever special arrangements are required for them to lead a dignified life, and the work of caring for them should be socially recognized, fairly distributed, and fairly compensated.

The "Dilemma of Difference"

In applying the capabilities approach to questions of provision for children with disabilities and special educational needs, Terzi (2005) engages with the dilemma of difference, which is the risk of reinforcing the stigma associated with assigned difference (such as an impairment) either by focusing on it, or by ignoring it (Minow 1985). To do the first is to risk labelling the person by calling attention to their difference from others; to do the latter is to risk not providing the enabling conditions that enable the person's quality of life. The dilemma of difference translated into institutional action involves having to choose from two equally problematic solutions in order to provide equitably for students with disabilities. The first option would be identifying the needs of students with disabilities and providing for them according to these needs, such as providing a university bus to take students with disabilities shopping because local taxis either will not transport them (if they have a guide dog), or charge double if they travel with a wheelchair. The bus is tremendously helpful but the individualized support marks the students out as different and does not address the need for policy changes. As Salais (2009) points out, the common good beyond the individual good would be best served by public policies which genuinely expand people's capabilities so that the real possibility of an alternate way of being exists, enabling "free access to a real possibility" (2009, 6). Another option would be to treat students as all the same and offer standardized provision. But this results in the failure to make relevant external provision, such as adapted student residences or additional learning support, for those who might require it for such "free access to a real possibility."

Using Sen as her reference point, Terzi (2005) argues that the capabilities approach can resolve the dilemma of difference. By reconsidering this dilemma through the freedoms and opportunities to do what one values, the capabilities approach moves beyond the dual framing of disability in the individual (stigmatize) or the social environment (treat all as equal) to a relational approach that considers both individual impairment and educational arrangements. It considers the specificity of a situation as well as each individual's agency. In this manner it avoids labelling people with disabilities based on their impairment only. Terzi further says that the capabilities approach highlights how the disability has to be addressed as a matter of social justice, since this contributes to the equalization of the individual's capability to achieve well-being (Terzi, 2005). Similarly, Nussbaum (2006) contends that social contract theory cannot bring justice to people with disabilities because the framework does not allow their full participation in activities they value. Social contract theories conceive that basic political principles as a result of reciprocity—a contract for mutual advantage. In this scheme, students with disabilities will suffer as they are not among those "for whom and in reciprocity with whom society's basic institutions are structured" (Nussbaum 2006, 98). For this reason, we align ourselves to Nussbaum's approach in having a specified list of capabilities (although we do not claim that our list is universal as Nussbaum does with her list) with which to judge how socially just higher education institutions are in action, with regards to students with disabilities.

A list of capabilities

One way of resolving the dilemma of difference within the capabilities framework is through the identification of a list of valued capabilities that are context specific. Disability within the capabilities approach is conceptualized in relation to individuals set of functionings and capabilities to choose and lead what they regard as "a good life" (Sen 2009, 56). Focusing on a list of capabilities for students with disabilities provides a way of not seeing differences pertaining to disability in stigmatizing or discriminatory ways by focusing on the opportunities of individuals instead of their impairments. As noted earlier, Nussbaum (2000, 35) makes a case for a list of 10 central capabilities arguing that, "certain universal norms of human capability should be central for political purposes in thinking about basic political principles that can provide the underpinning for a set of constitutional guarantees in all nations." We are attracted to the idea of visionary, capabilities-based norms to give "bite" to public disability policy and to adjudicate whether human dignity and social justice is being addressed. We do not, however, propose a universal and comprehensive list as Nussbaum does, nor do we rely only on theory in formulating a disabilities list. Rather we try also to pay attention to Sen's (1999) argument for contextual deliberative processes in the formulation of any list of capabilities through our research process grounded in student voices which, while not strictly deliberative in the fullest sense, takes seriously those voices and lives of people mostly affected by any disability policy. We do think that the identification of capabilities is important and that student provision should be designed accordingly. Policy evaluation to measure the progress of different higher education institutions would then be based on how they are performing against the list.

Various scholars have proposed lists of capabilities for different constituencies (see Nussbaum 2011; Walker 2006; Wilson-Strydom 2015; Wolff and de-Shalit 2007). Focusing on higher education and pedagogies, Walker (2006) argues that a capabilities list is important but it should be contextual, provisional and the product of ongoing public dialogue. Focusing on pedagogies, Walker (2006) developed a capabilities list for higher education by reviewing six existing capabilities lists (including Alkire 2002; Flores-Crespo 2004) and drew on empirical work with university students, together with her own experience working in higher education. It is from the descriptions of her capabilities list that we drew some of our interview schedule questions. We made use of Walker's (2006) higher education capabilities list as it shares the same higher education context as in this paper. In constructing the interview schedule and questions, we drew on Walker's eight capabilities (see Table 1). At the analysis stage the interviews were coded according to these capabilities. Additionally, we used the list by Wolff and De-Shalit (2007) who did empirical work to evaluate the value of Nussbaum's list. They expanded her list to add the following capabilities: (a) doing good to others, (b) living in a law-abiding fashion, (c) understanding the law and (d) the ability to understand and speak the local language. Below we give the background and methodology of this study.

Table 1. Questions derived from Walker's list

Walker's capabilities	Description from Walker (2006, 128–129)	Generated questions
1. Practical reason	"Being able to make well-reasoned, informed, critical, independent, intellectually acute, socially responsible, and reflective choices. Being able to construct a personal life project in an uncertain world. Having good judgement."	What are your reasons for taking the course you are studying? How did you choose your course of study? In what ways do you think university education is helping you or will help you in the future?
2. Educational resilience	"Able to navigate study, work and life. Able to negotiate risk, to persevere academically, to be responsive to educational opportunities and adaptive to constraints. Self-reliant. Having aspirations and hopes for a good future."	What are your personal characteristics and other external factors that help you in the university? What are your personal characteristics and other external factors that restrict you at times in your educational goals? How is getting around the university for you like? Where do you see yourself in the next five years?
3. Knowledge and imagination	"Being able to gain knowledge of a chosen subject. Being able to use critical thinking and imagination to comprehend the perspectives of multiple others and to form impartial judgements. Being able to acquire knowledge for pleasure and personal development, for career and economic opportunities, for political, cultural and social action and participation in the world. Open-mindedness."	Which course modules do you like most and why? In what ways do you think your course of study is preparing you for the working environment? Besides the working related knowledge, what are five major issues you have learnt from your course that are beneficial to your community? Describe how lecturers run classes. What do you like about the way they are run? What would you like lecturers to do differently?
4. Learning disposition	"Being able to have curiosity and a desire for learning. Having confidence in one's ability to learn. Being an active inquirer."	Who inspired you on your university endeavours? What skills are helping you to succeed in your studies?
5. Social relations and social networks	"Being able to participate in a group for learning, working with others to solve problems and tasks. Being able to work with others to form effective or good groups for collaborative and participatory learning. Being able to form networks of friendship and belonging for learning support and leisure. Mutual trust."	Have you changed a situation that affects you or other students here? In what ways do you support other students? Do you belong to any social club (in/out of class)? How do you feel at home and when you are here? Are you treated differently here compared to your home? How do you feel about group work/group assignments? How was it in creating friendships at this institution? Who are your friends in terms of gender, race or other identities? What is the attitude of your friends towards you?

(*Continued*)

Table 1. Continued.

Walker's capabilities	Description from Walker (2006, 128–129)	Generated questions
6. Respect, dignity and recognition	"Being able to have respect for oneself and for and from others, being treated with dignity, not being diminished or devalued because of one's gender, social class, religion or race, valuing other languages, other religions and spiritual practices and human diversity. Being able to act inclusively and being able to respond to human need. Having competence in intercultural communication. Being able to show empathy, compassion, fairness and generosity, listening to and considering other person's points of view in dialogue and debate. Having a voice to participate effectively in learning; a voice to speak out, to debate and persuade; to be able to listen."	What does disability mean to you? What does impairment mean to you? How do you perceive yourself? / Describe what it means to you to have a disability/ impairment? How do you think other students and lecturers perceive you? Can you comment on the language policy of this university?
7. Emotional integrity, emotions	"Not being subject to anxiety or fear which diminishes learning. Being able to develop emotions for imagination, understanding, empathy, awareness and discernment."	What is your greatest fear? How do you deal with it?
8. Bodily integrity	"Safety and freedom from all forms of physical and verbal harassment in the higher education environment."	Were you ever made to feel that you were different to others by an event or personalities within this institution (with reference to your body)? (verbally and/ physically)

Context and Methodology

Findings from this paper are derived from a large qualitative study that was conducted in South Africa at two universities from 2013 to 2015 in order to understand how students with disabilities negotiate different spaces within SAHE and the nuanced aspects of disability. We first provide sufficient detail to situate the two universities and their variations; in both cases the universities agreed to be named. The University of the Free State (UFS) is a historically advantaged White Afrikaans university[1] founded in 1904. With the advent of democracy in 1994 the university changed to parallel medium of communication offering both English and Afrikaans classes rather than only Afrikaans. The student population is now around 30 431 and is predominantly black (70%), and the university is undertaking various transformation projects aimed at improving diversity issues focused on race and reconciliation of black and white students. Both gender and disability feature weakly in relation to diversity. The second institution is the University of Venda (UniVen), a rural and historically disadvantaged university with almost 100% Black/African students. It was established under apartheid policy in the northern province of Limpopo in 1981 as a branch of the University of the North (now the University of Limpopo), to serve the Venda/African community. It became an independent university in 1982. Currently, it has a student population of 14 133. Resourcing by government pre-1994 was limited and even post 1994 has been slow to address the disparities between apartheid advantaged and disadvantaged universities.

In order to conduct the research, lists with names and contacts of registered students with disabilities at Disability Services Units (DSUs) were provided by the DSU staff. Although disability is conceptualized in the capabilities approach as capability deprivation, operationally in this paper, we define disability as based on impairment, and investigate capability deprivations among persons with impairments which we refer to as disabilities. Purposive sampling was used to recruit eligible participants via email and telephone. All eligible participants were given information about the study and those who volunteered signed a consent form. Six students did not wish to take part in the study, eight students at UFS and six students at UniVen agreed. Student participants were from different races, disability categories and their levels of education and programmes of study were also different. The names of the student participants have been anonymized to protect their identities. Interview questions were drawn from literature and the input from pilot study participants. Furthermore, Walker's (2006) capabilities descriptions were utilized to formulate questions to identify valued, achieved and deprived capabilities. In-depth interviews, field observations and document analysis were used to gather data from participants. Interviews lasted between 40 and 80 minutes and were used to gather personal experiences and perceptions about disability from all participants. Data were analysed thematically with the aid of NVivo software. Interviews were coded thematically using both emerging codes and predetermined codes for example, Walker's eight capabilities formed part of the codes. Besides Walker's capability dimensions as explained above, interviews were also coded using Wolff and de-Shalit's descriptions. Descriptions which we thought were not fitting to Walker (2006) and, Wolff and De-Shalit's (2007) lists were coded as additional higher education capabilities.

Findings

This section presents the findings of the study which are the capabilities which we derived from participants' valued functionings.

Capabilities and Valued Functionings

Various functionings were drawn from the interviews and matched to Walker and, Wolff and De-Shalit's lists thematically. In this section we discuss capabilities that emerged from participants' data. We first discuss capabilities from Walker's (2006) list, this will be followed by a discussion of the capabilities from Wolff and De-Shalit's (2007) list. The last section explores the capabilities that are not in Walker, nor in Wolff and de-Shalit's lists.

Capabilities from Walker's (2006) List

Educational Resilience

Educational resilience is one of the capabilities listed by Walker (2006). Participants showed remarkable resilience in their education experiences, despite overwhelming challenges generated by conversion factors. Most students practised educational resilience in order to secure their other valued capabilities. The quotation below provides an example of participants' resilience:

> When I have some problems and I go to some of my lecturers they say to me, "go to those people at the Unit for Students with Disabilities." I would say, "but you are my lecturer and you are supposed to help me." I avoid lecturers like that and work with those who understand me better ... At times when I want to do an assignment I go to the library to look for reading materials but I don't find the books I want for that particular assignment. So I go to the computer lab for the internet, but at times when I get there the internet will be down. (Sipho)

It is clear that resilience is important for example, in Sipho's case above. However, students with disabilities' educational resilience still needs to be complemented by guarantees of the opportunities they value; universities need to play their role in promoting and ensuring that all students are treated with dignity.

Knowledge and imagination

The capability of knowledge and imagination is about being able to gain knowledge in one's field of study. This involves knowledge for personal development, for career and economic opportunities, for political, cultural and social action and participation in society. This was highlighted by Lerato and Sipho:

> I appreciate the university environment and the people around because I have learnt a lot since I got here. I have become more independent, I am more aware of what the outside world holds. Within the university there are people who open your eyes to the possibilities of your future and what tomorrow holds. (Lerato)

> Before I enrolled for my degree in Development Studies, I did not know how people should respond when there are getting poor services from local authorities. Through the course I now know who to approach and I will take a lead when I go back to my community. (Sipho)

Acquisition of the capability of knowledge and imagination can occur where students' social relations are smooth and affiliation (respect and recognition in relationships) is present to build their confidence. Participants also value field or discipline related skills and knowledge. This is to be expected, given the fact that this is the reason why they enrolled for higher education. Alongside acquisition of knowledge and skills are other "beings and doings" that are equally important.

Respect, Dignity and Recognition

Most participants value being treated with respect. This capability is at the centre of what disabled students need to access and succeed in higher education.

> I think this university is nice. They don't look at you whether you are coming from a poor background. They are not particular about the way you dress-you wear what you want. (Pat)

> I have gradually adapted into the Deaf culture. I feel emotionally and psychologically supported and appreciated when I am amongst deaf people than when I am amongst non-sign language users. (Dudu)

> I once felt segregated. I was in a group for a group assignment and they said that there is no important contribution I could make. I was side-lined. Fortunately, I joined another group where I was accepted as a blind person who could make valuable contributions to the group. (Toni)

When the capability for respect, dignity and recognition is taken away from them by universities, some participants may give up on exercising their individual agency. This was exemplified during data collection when the first author spent a day with Ralph, a blind student, and accompanied him to classes. In one of the morning lectures the first author recorded a lecturer instructing students, "See … after page 5, you will see a Table with surface learning [approach] on one side and deep learning [approach] on the other side." No account was taken of any student unable to see the page. Later that evening, the first author accompanied Ralph to a different lecture (they were about 20 in the lecture room) where they sat at the front, closer to the lecturer. The lecturer played a movie clip and instructed students to watch it for a discussion afterwards. The first author was surprised because at no point did she seem to notice Ralph's presence yet they were seated very close to her. In both cases Ralph was not "seen" and not being seen was accorded neither respect nor recognition of his different identity, nor was any effort made to address his learning support needs. This is a good example of "same treatment" to all students by higher education institutions leading to very unfair service provision for students.

Social Relations and Social networks

The capability for social relations and social networks is linked to functionings such as being able to participate in a group at the university either for learning or pleasure. Having a network of friendships from varied backgrounds and being given the opportunities to create friendships within the university, which was also valued by participants:

> We [wheelchair users] only have access to two student residences on campus, our own and the one for female wheelchair users. It's wrong because it seems as if they are isolating us from the rest of the students. We want to socialise with others. (Musa)

> First year students have an orientation week full of activities where they build friendships within residences. So at the end of the induction week friendships and networks would have been created. As wheelchair users we were thrown in a senior residence as it was the only residence that was wheelchair friendly. However, senior residences are not involved in the orientation week activities. We felt unwelcomed at this university. We missed out during the orientation week. (Anna)

Participants value social relations and social networks highly, both during their transition into and during their period in the university. Unfortunately, both universities fell short in promoting this capability in relation to students with disabilities.

Four capabilities on Walker's list did not appear strongly in our analysis. These are practical reason, learning disposition, emotional integrity and bodily integrity. There are possible explanations for this. In some cases, participants' responses to the questions generated for one capability tended to speak more to other capabilities. For example, we could have coded Dudu's narrative about language capability under *bodily integrity* or *emotional integrity*, but given the context of our participants and how they are identified, this seemed to be speaking more to the *language* capability as described by Wolff and De-Shalit (2007). Most responses to the questions about emotional integrity and bodily integrity were often negative one word answers—no. Either participants had not thought about these issues or the phrasing of the questions was difficult to comprehend. Another reason might be that participants had adapted to the conditions which they would not have accepted in fair situations. These capabilities might not be their primary concerns compared to challenges associated with being identified as people with disabilities. Ralph's narrative further in the paper seems to suggest adaptive preference. With regards to *learning disposition*, participants showed "curiosity and desire for learning", in their narratives about how they made it to universities and how they "persevere academically" at the university. In this paper, this is captured under educational resilience as it highlights how they exercise their agency when faced with barriers that hinder them from securing their well-being. Resilience on the part of the students with disabilities should not be used to obscure the need to address the limitations of provision within these universities and the need to attend to practices that are unjust.

Capabilities from Wolff and De-Shalit's (2007) list

Language

A capability which falls outside Walker's list of capabilities but which is from Wolff and De-Shalit's (2007) list is the ability to understand and speak the local language. Wilson-Strydom (2015, 131) has a similar capability under her capabilities for university readiness. She highlights the importance of the language capability which she describes as "being able to understand, read, write and speak confidently in the language of instruction." For students at UFS, which uses both Afrikaans and English for teaching and learning, language competence is important to all students. Lerato sees language as suffused also by issues of race. Given that Afrikaans-speaking lecturers and students in these classes are predominantly or entirely white, or some lecturers lapse into using Afrikaans or explaining in Afrikaans in what is supposed to be an English medium class:

> There are also race issues within this university. Some lecturers have a tendency of conducting their lectures in Afrikaans. What if I don't understand Afrikaans? (Lerato)

What we see is again an overlap between respect (respecting each person's right to learn in either English or Afrikaans) and recognition (of all identities at the university, not privileging an Afrikaans identity over others), and that of language. At UniVen which uses only English for teaching and instruction, the capability for language was connected to cultural differences. According to Kudzi, some lecturers at UniVen are from the Venda community as are the majority of student population. Difficulties arise when Venda-speaking lecturers and students begin to converse in Venda in classes that are supposed to be taught in English.

For Dudu who is a sign language user, the absence of interpreters has an adverse impact on his life at the university:

> I did nursing at the Free State school of Nursing after I resigned from the army. I only passed my first year. It required a lot of effort because there were no interpreters. I eventually left in the second year just because it was hectic, no interpreters to facilitate. I went home until I met that guy who advised me to apply to this university. (Dudu)

His case reveals that not only does the capability of language competence and confidence encompass being able to understand, read, write and speak confidently in the language of instruction but also being able to access knowledge in a language that is accessible to students, for example, sign language, and respecting student diversity.

Additional Higher Education Capabilities

Students' narratives show that there are some capability descriptions that we think can be foregrounded to stand as important capabilities for students with disabilities.

Aspiration

The capability to aspire also emerged from the data as significant opportunities and skills that can be fostered (Gaspar and Van Staveren 2003) in higher education.

> … in my family no one has had the motivation to go and study further. Being a third child, with my elder brothers struggling to get jobs with their Matric qualifications and all of us being raised by a single parent with a Grade 11 certificate and couldn't get a permanent stable job so I declared that I want a different lifestyle. I want to get a proper job and work, be able to earn my own money and have my own home. I don't want to be counted among those who receive a disability grant. Some of my classmates would say that they are content with a disability grant but I would say it won't be always enough for me to cater for everything I need. One day I will need a house, my own house. I can't live at my mother's house forever. And also the fact that my mother passed away when I was 14 and since I never knew my father you know it was just basically me and my brothers so I felt I am responsible of taking care of my younger sister. I just said let me just do the university thing. (Lerato)

> I am studying for my degree so that I can have a proper job one day. For me this is the most important thing of being in higher education because I want to be independent. I don't want to be dependent on my parents for the rest of my life. (Joe)

Unlike the view that positions some students as lacking aspiration, these findings highlight that capacities to articulate and pursue aspirations are affected by and affect other capabilities.

Culture

The capability to live without being tripped by culture also emerged strongly. It was thus not unexpected that with the exception of Toni, students did not refer to themselves as "disabled," or "with disabilities." This might be partly due to the negative cultural and societal beliefs towards disability or disabled people. When reference was made to the concepts, *disability* or *with disabilities* it was to answer that they were not identifiable with those labels.

Students explained their culture's views regarding people with impairments:

> The Pedi culture view visual impairment as a curse from God or ancestors as a result of my parents/ family's involvement in witchcraft act. (Toni)

> I think my parents took me there [special school] because people in the community were calling me names when I was still young. (Pat)

These strong culturally linked definitions came out only at UniVen. This could be a result of the fact that all interviewed students at UniVen come from rural communities, unlike those at UFS who come from urbanized communities where traditional cultures might not be as strong as in rural communities.

Identity

Being able to choose one's identity is one capability which emerged strongly in the interviews with students with disabilities. They expressed a dislike of the negative identities that are used to define them:

> To me it [disability] doesn't really mean anything. It's not how I see myself. It doesn't define me but people tend to categorise me with that label e.g. I am rarely introduced as "Lerato the law student," it's usually "Lerato, the disabled law student" or "Lerato the disabled student" or something along these lines. Some people like to see it [disability] as a term to define your obstacles e.g. the fact that I am in a wheelchair makes it okay for other people to say that I have a disability, I am differently abled or any other term they happen to come across. I am not disabled I am me. I am Lerato. I am just like any other person … you know I go through the same things that you go through the only thing that is different is that I use a wheelchair. (Lerato)

Being valued and being respected underpin Lerato's wanting to be able to define who she is for herself, not to be labelled by others, or to be defined by her disability. Lerato sees herself caught up in a dilemma. She does not see herself as a disabled student, yet she is registered as such with the DSU so as to receive support. We also see resilience at work and social relationships in a form here which Lerato does not value from which we can extrapolate the kind of social relations she does value.

Mobility

Being able to move from one place to another within the university was highlighted as important. We can extrapolate this from Lerato:

> The university knows that they have students who use wheelchairs. Surprisingly, some lectures and exams are scheduled in rooms where there are stairs and no lifts. We are forced to go to the lecturers who in turn have to arrange with the people who organise exam venues. At times it takes more than a week for corrective measures to be found and all this time you will be missing classes. Once you fall behind it's really hard to catch up. It's one thing that is not changing at this university.

The presence of an accessible higher education environment allows ease of access to offices, classrooms and residences.

Religion

Religion featured in students' narratives as contributing to their survival in difficult times:

> The bible sometimes consoles me at times. I feel good about the way I am because there are some comforting messages in it that we are all created in the image of God. Even some of the songs we sing at church, they sooth the soul. (Musa)

> I'm a ZCC [Zion Christian Church] member. Here on campus we congregate as members and advise one another and practice our religion. We are treated equally at church. (Toni)

Voice

In Walker's list of capabilities, voice as a capability is part of the respect, dignity and recognition capability. However, having a voice to participate effectively in the university, individually or collectively, emerged strongly warranting it as a separate capability:

> I mobilised other disabled students when we were having persistent challenges at our residence. We decided to skip all the bureaucracy and we went straight to the university Rector. We sat down with the Rector and we highlighted our concerns. Since then a lot has improved because now when we have problems we approach the Rector directly. (Lerato)

> As disabled students we have our own Disabled Student Representative Council. We always push our chairperson to represent us well when he meets the university management. (Musa)

Lerato is resilient, has a voice and is an agent, and her resilience and voice are crucial to this agency—she does not give up in the face of adversity, she bounces back, she is determined. Again we see how one capability strengthens another and how capabilities are necessary for agency and how students mobilize their voices together through their own Council to get what they collectively value. We now turn to the discussion section.

Discussion

A set of basic capabilities valued by students with disabilities in SAHE were extrapolated. Although this was a small-scale study and further studies are needed, nonetheless paying attention to these capabilities for both students with disabilities and those without disabilities within higher education should be a necessity for policy. For students with disabilities in SAHE to have access to an education that allows them to flourish, equal opportunities should be made available to them.

A list of capabilities is useful in resolving the problem of dilemma of difference. Instead of focusing on human differences, policies would be targeted at freedoms and opportunities that support the identified capabilities and no capabilities will be overlooked through omission (Nussbaum 2000). It is arguably easier if we do not have a list of capabilities to provide information to policy-makers for policies to overlook those who might have adapted their preference under bad circumstances (for example, resigning themselves as Ralph does to being ignored by his lecturers and hence possibly not mentioning the need for lecturer support). Moreover, when we have a list of capabilities, there will be no excuse on the part of powerful institutions like universities to deny marginalized people their valued opportunities and freedoms. Programmes, pedagogies and curriculum can be designed accordingly to foster these identified capabilities.

This list of capabilities also confirms that valuable capabilities are context specific. Four of Walker's capabilities which emerged out of international higher education with diverse student populations are applicable to students with disabilities in the global South. These findings are important in challenging the idea of treating students with disabilities strictly as a separate group from other students. There is a danger of obscuring areas of commonality that exist between the experiences of students with disabilities and students without disabilities. It would be more beneficial to students with disabilities for higher education to concentrate on cultivating the identified capabilities than dwelling only on the difference between students with disabilities and students without disabilities, precisely because capabilities in their conceptualization avoids the dilemma of difference trap. Of course a capabilities list also raises the need for tradeoffs in the provision of services for a diverse student population. Not all capabilities from Walker's list emerged strongly from these students with disabilities' narratives. *Emotional integrity and emotions; bodily integrity*, and *Practical reason* did not feature much. This might suggest that students with disabilities in higher education have other different valued capabilities to those of students without disabilities, yet what they value is equally important to any student. Another reason might be our own interpretation of the data as researchers. Walker (2006) notes that there are elements within her capabilities descriptions which might be foregrounded by other scholars as capabilities. For example, the capability for *identity* might be considered by others as fitting under the capability for *respect, dignity and recognition*.

This study is also important in assessing the significance of the capabilities approach in the fields of higher education and disability. While scholars have come up with different ways of establishing capabilities, we have shown here, through our analysis of the narratives with an existing list that there is no single "correct" approach in coming up with a list of capabilities. As our data show, most students with disabilities lack opportunities and freedoms to secure their capabilities. In responding to the SDGs debates, higher education institutions and policy-makers ought to pay attention to institutional policies which determine actions and non-actions that negatively affect students with disabilities' opportunities to secure: *aspiration; educational resilience; cultural value; choice of identity; knowledge and imagination; language; mobility; religious affiliation; respect dignity and recognition; social relations and social networks and voice*. This might be achieved through induction programmes on inclusive and diversity issues for staff and more resources. As for the general student population, this calls for the fostering of extra-curriculum, curriculum and pedagogical practices which celebrate differences and commonalities, and which develop student awareness, empathy and action with regard to the lives of students with disabilities.

Findings highlight the multi-dimensionality at work in that capabilities enhanced other capabilities, so that, for example, the capability of *knowledge and imagination* is closely related to the capability for *social relations and social networks*; they reinforce each other.

Each capability should be incommensurable, but one or two may be architectonic. It is apparent in the analysis of these identified capabilities that the capability to *aspire* and *respect, dignity and recognition* seem to be the key capabilities which enable the realization of other capabilities. These capabilities have multiplier effects. Treating someone with respect involves according someone identities that are not devalued or demeaning, and further having the ability to choose one's *identity*. It also means recognizing one's *language* with the same priority as other languages. With these in place, *social relations and social networks* can be easily promoted, enhancing the capability of *voice* which ultimately promotes *educational resilience* leading to the acquisition of *knowledge and skills* in higher education.

Conclusion

This paper deepens, and expands ongoing conversations on disability in higher education and within the capabilities approach. It applies the capabilities approach to the specific case of students with disabilities in higher education. Eleven capabilities were extrapolated: *aspiration; educational resilience; cultural value; choice of identity; knowledge and imagination; language; mobility; religious affiliation; respect dignity and recognition; social relations and social networks and voice*. These capabilities advance the capabilities approach by being specific to students with disabilities and focusing on higher education.

We have argued that the relevant valued functionings identified by students with disabilities are not distributed fairly in and through SAHE. In this instance, the capabilities approach directs attention to salient features of inequalities in higher education that perpetuate social injustice. Additionally, the approach provides a persuasive analysis of issues and enables recommendations for action. Higher education and disability policy-makers can question the extent to which each one is being promoted or inhibited within and across different higher education institutions. This data makes it possible to move beyond evaluating educational outcomes based only on student graduation rates and exam performance. It enables one to measure the gap between the lived experiences of students and what they value in higher education. This is one of the ways which shows the significance of the capabilities approach compared to other disability models. The exercise of individual agency and choice (which is overlooked by other disability models) is important in these students' lives. Ultimately, these capabilities can be taken up pedagogically, instituted in higher education, and secured to students with disabilities through embedding them in the curriculum and in institutions.

Acknowledgements

We acknowledge the valuable comments and suggestions from Sophie Mitra, anonymous peer reviewers and the funding support to the CRHED by the UFS and the National Research Fund for this study.

Disclosure statement

No potential conflict of interest was reported by the authors.

Notes

1. Under apartheid, higher education institutions were designed to serve only one of the four apartheid racial groups (Africans, Coloureds, Indians and Whites). Broadly speaking, White universities were advantaged in terms of their resourcing, and Black universities disadvantaged, with fewer resources and students coming from poor schooling backgrounds.
2. Pseudonym.
3. These are the categories into which participants fall as defined by the universities.
4. Coloured is an ethnic label for people of mixed origin who possess ancestry from Europe, Asia, and various Khoisan and Bantu-speaking tribes of Southern Africa.

References

Alkire, S. 2002. *Valuing Freedoms. Sen's Capability Approach and Poverty Reduction*. Oxford: Oxford University Press.

Alkire, S. 2008. "Choosing Dimensions: The Capability Approach and Multidimensional Poverty." In *The Many Dimensions of Poverty*, edited by N. Kakwani and J. Silber, 89–119. New York: Palgrave Macmillan.

Barnes, C., and G. Mercer. 2003. *Disability*. Cambridge: The Polity Press.

Bury, M. 2000. "On Chronic Illness and Disability." In *Handbook of Medical Sociology*, edited by C. E. Bird, P. Conrad and A. M. Fremont, 173–184. 5th ed. New Jersey, PA: Prentice Hall.

Department of Higher Education and Training (DHET). 2013. "White Paper on Post-school Education and Training." Retrieved from http://www.dhet.gov.za/SiteAssets/Latest%20News/White%20paper%20for%20post-school%20education%20and%20training.pdf.

Flores-Crespo, P. 2004. "Situating Education in the Human Capabilities Approach." Paper presented at the Fourth Conference on the Capability Approach: Enhancing Human Security, Pavia, Italy.

Fuller, M., and M. Healey. 2009. "Assessing Disabled Students: Student and Staff Experiences of Reasonable Adjustments." In *Improving Disabled Students' Learning*, edited by M. Fuller, J. Georgeson, M. Healey, A. Hurst, K. Kelly, S. Riddell, H. Roberts, and E. Weedon, 40–78. London: Routledge.

Gaspar, D., and I. Van Staveren. 2003. "Development as Freedom – And as What Else?" *Feminist Economics* 9 (2–3): 137–161.
Minow, M. 1985. "Learning to Live with the Dilemma of Difference: Bilingual and Special Education." *Law and Contemporary Problems* 48 (2): 157–211.
Mitra, S. 2006. "The Capability Approach and Disability." *Journal of Disability Policy Studies* 16: 236–247.
Mitra, S. 2014. "Reconciling the Capability Approach and the ICF: A Response." *ALTER – European Journal of Disability Research* 8 (1): 24–29.
Mitra, Sophie, A. Posarac, and B. Vick. 2013. "Disability and Poverty in Developing Countries: A Multidimensional Study." *World Development* 41: 1–18.
Nussbaum, M. C. 2000. *Women and Human Development: The Capabilities Approach*. Cambridge: Cambridge University Press.
Nussbaum, M. 2006. *Frontiers of Justice: Disability, Nationality, Species Membership*. Cambridge, MA: Belknap Press.
Nussbaum, M. 2011. *Creating Capabilities: The Human Development Approach*. Cambridge, MA: The Belknap Press.
Oliver, M. 1996. *Understanding Disability: From Theory to Practice*. London: Macmillan.
Reindal, S. M. 2009. "Disability, Capability, and Special Education: Towards a Capability-based Theory." *European Journal of Special Needs Education* 24 (2): 155–168.
Salais, R. 2009. "Deliberative Democracy and its Informational Basis: What Lessons from the Capability Approach." Society for the Advancement of Socio-Economics Conference, Paris, France.
Sen, A. 1999. *Development as Freedom*. New York: Knopf.
Sen, A. 2009. *The Idea of Justice*. London: Penguin.
Shakespeare, T. 2014. *Disability Rights and Wrongs Revisited*. London: Routledge.
Strnadova, I., V. Hájková, and L. Květoňová. 2015. "Voices of University Students with Disabilities: Inclusive Education on the Tertiary Level – A Reality or a Distant Dream?" *International Journal of Inclusive Education*. doi:10.1080/13603116.2015.1037868.
Terzi, L. 2005. "Beyond the Dilemma of Difference: The Capability Approach to Disability and Special Educational Needs." *Journal of Philosophy of Education* 39: 443–459.
Terzi, L. 2010. *Justice and Equality in Education: A Capability Perspective on Disability and Special Educational Needs*. London: Continuum.
Trani, J., P. Bakhshi, N. Bellanca, M. Biggeri, and F. Marchetta. 2011. "Disabilities Through the Capability Approach Lens: Implications for Public Policies." *ALTER – European Journal of Disability Research / Revue Européenne de Recherche sur le Handicap* 5 (3): 143–157.
Trani, J. F., and T. Cannings. 2013. "Child Poverty in an Emergency and Conflict Context: A Multidimensional Profile and an Identification of the Poorest Children in Western Darfur?" *World Development* 48: 48–70.
Unterhalter, E. 2003. "Crossing Disciplinary Boundaries: The Potential of Sen's Capability Approach for Sociologists of Education." *British Journal of Sociology of Education* 24 (5): 665–669.
Vickerman, P., and M. Blundell. 2010. "Hearing the Voices of Disabled Students in Higher Education." *Disability & Society* 25 (1): 21–32.
Walker, M. 2006. *Higher Education Pedagogies: A Capabilities Approach*. Maidenhead: Society for Research on Higher Education/ Open University Press and McGraw-Hill.
Warnock, M., B. Norwich, and L. Terzi, eds. 2010. *Special Educational Needs: A New Look*. London: Continuum International Publishing Group.
Wilson-Strydom, M. 2015. *University Access and Success: Capabilities, Diversity and Social Justice*. New York: Routledge.
Wolff, J., and A. De-Shalit. 2007. *Disadvantage*. Oxford: Oxford University Press.

Appendix

Participants' profile

Name[2]	Institution	Category[3]	Age	Faculty	Gender	Race
Kudzi	UniVen	Partially sighted	39	Education	Female	Black
Pat	UniVen	Other-Albinism	30	Human and Social Sciences	Female	Black
Musa	UniVen	Physical disability	29	Law	Male	Black
Sipho	UniVen	Partially sighted	21	Human and Social Sciences	Male	Black
Mpho	UniVen	Physical disability	22	Law	Male	Black
Toni	UniVen	Blind	28	Human and Social Sciences	Male	Black
Carla	UFS	Learning disability-Dyslexia	22	Economic and Management Sciences	Female	Coloured[4]
Lerato	UFS	Physical disability	25	Law	Female	Black
Anna	UFS	Physical disability	25	Law	Female	Black
Jane	UFS	Other-Epileptic	20	The Humanities	Female	White
Joe	UFS	Blind	26	The Humanities	Male	White
Ralph	UFS	Blind	18	Education	Male	Coloured
Michael	UFS	Physical disability	18	Education	Male	Black
Dudu	UFS	Hearing	38	The Humanities	Male	Black

Disability and Poverty in Morocco and Tunisia: A Multidimensional Approach

JEAN-FRANCOIS TRANI, PARUL BAKHSHI, SARAH MYERS TLAPEK, DOMINIQUE LOPEZ & FIONA GALL

ABSTRACT *Although a growing body of research is exploring the links between disability and poverty, the evidence that persons with disabilities are more likely to be poor than their non-disabled counterpart remains scarce. The causal relationship between disability and poverty has most often been considered in terms of disparities in income or living conditions. However, some research strongly suggests that disability is associated with deprivation in a number of other dimensions. To date, no study has examined these associations using large scale surveys with a wide range of wellbeing dimensions and indicators using a multidimensional approach. The present paper presents findings of three multidimensional poverty measures based on 17 indicators of deprivation collected through large-scale household surveys in Morocco and Tunisia. These indicators cover a wide range of dimensions of poverty such as health, education, employment, material well-being, social participation, psychological well-being and physical security. Results confirm that persons with disabilities are poorer than non-disabled people in both countries. The study shows that persons with disabilities, particularly girls and women, rural residents, and those with intellectual, mental or multiple disabilities are particularly deprived of basic capabilities and functionings and that stigma plays a role in this social injustice. Civil society organizations should take the lead to promote awareness of social and emotional well-being of persons with disabilities.*

1. Introduction

After decades of limited research, there has recently been more interest among scholars in examining issues pertaining to disability in low- and middle-income countries (LMIC). Some studies have investigated access to essential services including education and health care (Filmer 2008; Trani et al. 2011); others have explored the disparities in access to employment and wage gaps (Mitra and Sambamoorthi 2009; Mizunoya and Mitra 2013). Finally, general living conditions have also been the object of examination in LMICs (Eide and Loeb 2006; Trani, Bakhshi, and Dubois 2006).

Several recent studies in diverse settings provide evidence on the additional costs incurred by households with a member with disability. In India, Erb and Harris-White (2001) estimated three categories of costs associated with disability: a direct cost; an opportunity cost related to loss of income; and an indirect cost linked to the care provided by a caregiver. In Kenya and Yemen, Ingstad and Grut (2006, 2007) found an adverse impact on livelihoods of families with a disabled child (Grut and Ingstad 2006; Ingstad and Grut 2007). A small but growing body of studies in low- and middle-income settings demonstrate that persons with disabilities and their families are more often poorer and may be at higher risk of poverty than families who do not live with a disabled person (Filmer 2008; Mont and Cuong 2011; Trani and Loeb 2012; Mitra, Posarac, and Vick 2013; Trani and Cannings 2013).

The research on disability and poverty has recently been influenced by the work of Amartya Sen and the capability approach. Following Sen (1981, 1999), many scholars have argued that deprivation of basic capabilities, such as access to clean water, nutrition, shelter, education, health care and physical safety among others is a concern for social justice. Within the capability approach, social justice is closely linked to equality and "well-being freedom"; progress toward achieving justice is measured through an increase in the capability set (Barclay 2012; Drydyk 2012). An examination of the state of deprivation in basic capabilities requires a multidimensional poverty lens (Chiappero-Martinetti and Moroni 2007). This lens allows for scrutiny of inequalities in the capabilities of persons with disabilities and provides a comprehensive framework for examining the barriers to full participation in society (Trani et al. 2011). In recent years, several authors have developed measures of multidimensional poverty (Chiappero-Martinetti 2000; Bourguignon and Chakravarty 2003; Alkire and Foster 2011). Some have used multidimensional poverty measures to better understand issues related to disability, but have focused either on children (Trani, Biggeri, and Mauro 2013; Trani and Cannings 2013), or on adults in a limited set of middle- and low-income settings (Mitra, Posarac, and Vick 2013). Mitra et al. (2013) found that adults with disabilities have a higher likelihood of being multidimensionally poor than non-disabled adults, but the data include only 5 dimensions with 10 indicators. Trani, Biggeri, and Mauro (2013) and Trani and Cannings (2013) use data on more dimensions of well-being, but their results are specific to children in emergency or post-conflict contexts (Darfur and Afghanistan). The contribution of the present study is to provide the first population-level estimates of multidimensional poverty across disability status in two middle-income countries with a measure covering a wide range of well-being dimensions.

In 2013 and 2014, we carried out a case–control randomized household survey in Morocco and Tunisia, covering two geographical regions in each country. The household survey was taken from a representative sample of the diversity of the country. In the survey, we screened for disability and consequently interviewed identified persons with disabilities and non-disabled controls, matching by gender, age and area of residence. We subsequently examined poverty by applying the methodology developed by Alkire and Foster (2011), comparing the situation of persons with and without disabilities using three different measures of multidimensional poverty. Findings show that persons with disabilities face a higher level and intensity of multidimensional poverty in both countries. The study's findings have implications for policies aimed to improve the circumstances of persons with disabilities in both countries. Following the introduction, Section 2 of this paper briefly investigates the legal and political context of disability in Morocco and Tunisia and introduces the multidimensional approach to poverty. Section 3 describes the data collection process as well as measures for disability and multidimensional poverty. Section 4 presents findings and Section 5 discusses implications.

2. Background

2.1. Disability in Morocco and Tunisia

A national-level policy focus on disability is relatively recent in Morocco. The first law in 1982 targeted social protection for the visually impaired, and in 1993, the country adopted a general law addressing all disabilities. The country signed and ratified the United Nations Convention on the Rights of Persons with Disabilities (UNCRPD) in 2008. A 2004 national study on disability reported that 5.1% of the Moroccan population, around 1.53 million people, was living with a disability; one in four households. Access to health services was found to be a major problem for 55.3% of persons with disabilities, and another 52.5% coveted financial support to cover their basic needs (Secrétariat d'Etat chargé de la famille 2004). Only 13% of persons with disabilities, registered with the National Social Security Administration, were insured or received social assistance of any kind; among these, only 11% stated that their insurance covered all of their expenses. Nearly three-quarters of persons with disabilities of working age had no income-generating activity. Efforts are still needed to ensure that laws and their underlying principles are implemented at the levels of legislation, public policy and social practice. There is still widespread belief in Morocco that persons with disabilities are severely limited in their productive capacity and represent a burden on their families and a 'tax' on society as whole (Bakhshi et al. 2014a).

Tunisia has a longer history of addressing disability, with legislation in the 1960s establishing early structures for the care of persons with disabilities. However, the lack of consensus around definitions of disability and estimates of prevalence has limited the quality of needs assessment and hindered the design of effective strategies to meet identified needs (Chapireau 2002; Hamonet and Magalhaes 2003). A new law established in 2005 and the ratification of the UNCRPD (United Nations 2006) in 2008 have created a new impetus for promoting disability rights. Yet, Tunisia's disability policies and social norms remain rooted in a paradigm that views persons with disabilities as 'unfortunate charity-cases' who require care. The definition of disability outlined in the Tunisian legislation is not fully consistent with rights defined in the UNCRPD. People with intellectual disabilities and those with mental disorders are limited in their access to the disability card and basic services. Data on disability were extremely limited until the present study. The general population census of 1994 estimated the number of disabled persons at 1.2% of the total population, which is significantly lower than the findings from the present study, which estimates prevalence of severe disability at 5.7% (Bakhshi et al. 2014b).

3. Methodology

3.1. Sampling and Data Collection Process

We carried out two surveys in Morocco and Tunisia using the same methodology. We selected two geographical regions in each country which were representative of the diversity of the country in terms of urbanization, cultural and socioeconomic background. These include the regions of Rabat-Salé and Chaouia-Ouardhiga in Morocco, and the governorate of Tunis and Béja in Tunisia. Within each region, we used Moroccan and Tunisian census data from 2004 and 2001 respectively to randomly select clusters proportional to population

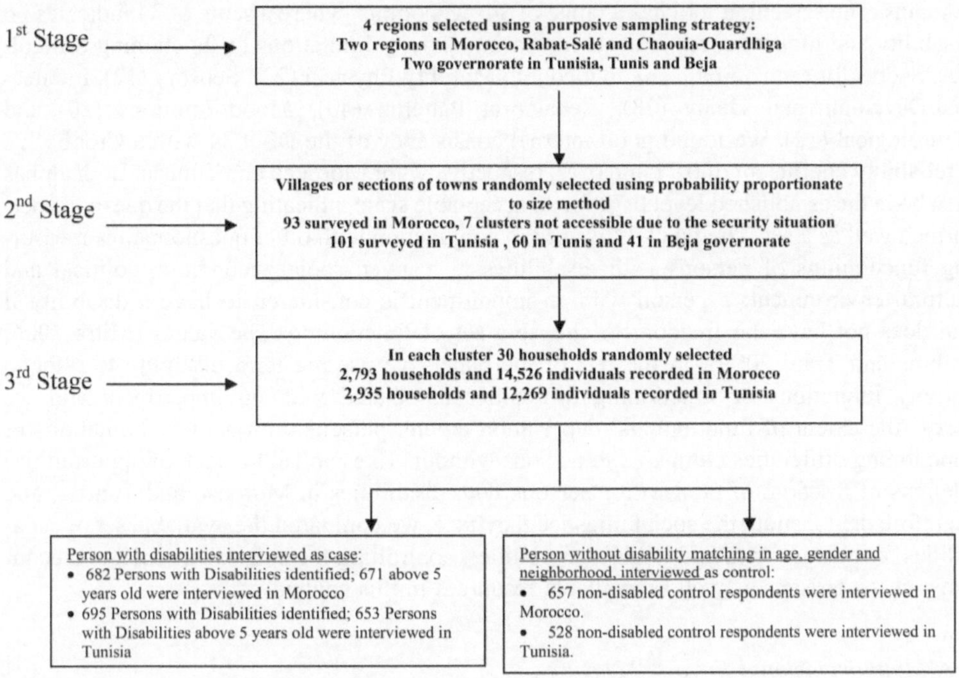

Figure 1. Sampling stages of the Moroccan and Tunisian case–control study.

size for a total of 194 clusters in both countries. Within each cluster, we randomly selected 30 households (See Figure 1 in Appendix).

The research team partnered with local experts on disability as well as representatives of Disabled Persons Organizations (DPOs) to develop the questionnaire after extensive consultation and formative qualitative research between August and October 2013. The team tested the questionnaire's content validity using focus groups discussions (FGDs) and in-depth interviews. The questionnaire was composed of two household modules including characteristics of the household, a disability-screening questionnaire (DSQ) and five individual modules (six modules in Tunisia) focusing on topics such as health, education and employment.

The data were collected between the November 4, 2013 and the February 8, 2014 successively in both countries. Enumerators administered household modules one and two to selected 2793 and 2935 heads of household in Morocco and Tunisia, respectively. The team conducted interviews using the individual modules in Morocco and Tunisia with 682 and 695 respondents with disabilities and 657 and 528 non-disabled respondents, respectively.

3.2. Disability Measure

The DSQ used in the present study is composed of 34 questions that were defined based on the International Classification of Functioning, Disability and Health (ICF) and were framed within the capability approach, allowing for identification of overall activity limitations and functioning difficulties in activities of daily living associated with an impairment (Trani and Bakhshi 2008). Developed in 2004 in Afghanistan, the DSQ-34 has since been validated and used in various LMICs settings (India, Nepal, Sierra Leone and Sudan). The DSQ-34 gives both a raw total score for disability and specific scores for each of the six domains. The screening tool has a range of 34–134 points, where a score of 34 indicates no disability and higher scores indicate increasing activity limitations or functioning difficulties. Scores for each domain are divided into Mobility/Physical (22), Sensory (12), Intellectual/Developmental Delay (28), Behavioral Patterns (40), Mood/Emotions (20) and Neurological (12). We found good internal consistency of the DSQ-34 with a Cronbach's α reliability coefficient of 0.71 and 0.77, respectively, for Morocco and Tunisia. Both alphas are above the established level 0.70 for an acceptable scale indicating that the questions performed well as a set. The DSQ-34 is used in conjunction with other questionnaires measuring functionings of persons with disabilities in a given social, economic, political and cultural environment: a person with an impairment is considered to have a disability if she does not have the freedom to choose a set of functionings she values (Mitra 2006; Dubois and Trani 2009). In the rest of the paper, we use the term disability to refer to activity limitations or functioning difficulties associated with an impairment and we assess the extent of functionings' deprivation among persons with activity limitations or functioning difficulties compared to persons without. To establish the lack of opportunities (deficits of freedom of choice) for persons with disabilities in Morocco and Tunisia, and therefore demonstrate the social injustice they face, we compared the available set of capabilities for persons with and without disabilities, controlling for individual social and economic characteristics as well as available resources in this context.

3.3. Multidimensional Poverty Measure

Multidimensional approaches to measuring poverty were developed in response to the critique that income alone does not suffice to determine poverty and that the concept of well-being includes multiple dimensions of human development. There are several benefits to a multidimensional approach, which not only allows for a more precise evaluation of human development policies but also creates a space for groups targeted by policies to shape definitions of poverty (Alkire 2002). Under the capability framework, the various dimensions of human development within a poverty measure should be either actual components of an individual's well-being, or they should have instrumental value for well-being (Sen 1999). A multidimensional poverty measure also needs to account for two central notions of poverty: who the poor are (what defines an individual as poor) and how many people within a population can be described as poor (Sen 1976, 1979, Sen 1981). Within this multidimensional perspective of human development and poverty, Alkire and Foster outlined a 'dual cutoff' method with two advantages: the first cut-off allows for analysis of poverty according to each dimension, and the second cut-off allows for a context-specific definition of poverty and the establishment of a 'multidimensional poverty level' that reflects public socio-political views (Alkire and Foster 2011).

This approach to measuring poverty falls along a spectrum of multidimensional measures. At one end of this spectrum is the "union method" which defines people as poor if they fall below desired levels in any one of the dimensions of poverty (Tsui 2002; Bourguignon and Chakravarty 2003; Deutsch and Silber 2005). At the opposite end of the spectrum is the "intersection method" in which the poor are described as those who fall below minimal levels in all dimensions of poverty.

Using Alkire and Foster (2011), we measured three indicators of multidimensional poverty: (i) the poverty headcount (H) which indicates how many individuals are found below the poverty line; (ii) the average deprivation share (A), which shows the average number of dimensions of deprivation endured by each poor person; and (iii) the adjusted headcount ratio (M_0), which is the product of the poverty rate (H) and the average deprivation share (A) and indicates the extent and intensity of poverty.

3.4. Selection of Dimensions and Cut-offs

The choice of dimensions was made via a participatory discussion process to adequately frame the issues within the specific cultural, social and economic contexts of Morocco and Tunisia (Alkire 2008; Mitra et al. 2013). Undeniably, the definition of basic capabilities and the threshold for access vary according to the context (Robeyns 2003). Seventeen indicators of essential functionings and corresponding basic capabilities were identified through an extensive literature review and validated through FGDs with persons with disabilities and experts in both countries. Participants came to a consensus with regard to the importance of factors of inequality and social exclusion (e.g. problems of access to quality health care, education, employment and shelter) and the crucial negative influence of stigmatizing behavior from community members. The 17 indicators which are considered essential components of well-being fall mainly within 7 dimensions of human development: health (2 indicators), education (2 indicators), employment (1 indicator), material well-being (6 indicators), social participation (2 indicators), psychological well-being (2 indicators) and physical security (2 indicators) (see Table 1).

The first dimension selected through the participatory process is health. Health is a basic capability; having the opportunity to achieve good health is essential to human development and is inherently linked to concerns of social justice (Sen 2002). Health is measured by access to quality health care and daily food intake. Unlike many low-income countries, Morocco and Tunisia have relatively accessible healthcare systems. Most persons with disabilities and non-disabled people report being able to access a healthcare facility (92.5% of persons with disabilities and controls report access to a healthcare facility). Yet, access to health care does not necessarily provide adequate treatment. A majority of respondents complained of the poor quality of health care provided, identifying long waiting times, high costs for drugs and tests, unavailability of needed devices, uncertain diagnosis and a lack of respect and courtesy from medical staff during interactions with patients. An essential basic capability of health was adequate nourishment, measured here as daily food intake (Alkire and Santos 2014). Nutrition is considered an essential indicator of development and constitutes the subject of the first millennium development goal. Morocco and Tunisia have made considerable progress since Independence in reducing undernutrition, but our study shows that access to food remains an issue of concern.

The second dimension identified was education. For adults, the first cut-off indicator of education was completion of primary education. Current enrollment in school was the cut-off for school-age children. Ability to read and write was the second cut-off indicator for both age groups. These thresholds correspond to Objective #2 outlined in the Millennium Development Goals: access to the full cycle of primary school. The role of education as a process for fighting discrimination, promoting social justice and overcoming poverty has been extensively illustrated in the literature. In particular, scholars have argued that education plays several roles. First, education plays an instrumental economic role in supporting employment. Second, education has a non-economic instrumental role in enhancing the capacity of the educated citizenry for critical thinking and public debate. Third, education has an instrumental role in promoting an expanded individual social network and allowing more interaction with others. Finally, it has an empowering role through the potential for political organization of the poor and the marginalized (Freire 1970; Robeyns 2006).

Non-employment is a major source of vulnerability for persons with disabilities both in High-Income Countries (HICs) and LMICs (Mitra and Sambamoorthi 2008; Gartrell 2010; Benoit et al. 2013; Mizunoya and Mitra 2013) and this was confirmed by respondents during the FGDs (Bakhshi et al. 2014a, b). Adults complained of the lack of opportunities in both countries and felt discouraged in their search for a job. Accordingly, poverty on this

Table 1. Dimensions of poverty and indicators of deprivation

Dimension	Indicators	Questions	Deprivation cut-off
1. Health	Quality of health care	Are you satisfied with the medical care/treatment you receive?	Not totally unsatisfied
	Food security	Do you get enough to eat?	Often or never enough to eat
2. Education	Adult educational attainment/children attendance	Did you go/Are you currently going to school?	Primary school incomplete for adults or not in school for school age children
	Literacy (read and write)	Do you know how to read and write?	Not able to read and write
3. Employment	Non-employment	Are you working?	Not working (only those 18–65 years)
4. Household-level material well-being	Access to clean drinking water	What is the main source of drinking water in your household?	Public tap, well, spring water, water tank
	Indoor air pollution	What is the main energy source used in your household for cooking?	Wood, kerosene and charcoal
	Type of toilet	What type of toilet facilities are used by your household?	Public toilets, septic system with or without ventilation, open air defecation
	Type of lighting	What is the main source of lighting in your household?	Generator, candle, oil lamp, anything other than electricity
	Overcrowding space	How many people are living together in your household?	More than three people per room
	Number and type of assets	Do you own the following items? Mobile phone, fixed telephone line, radio, refrigerator, electric fan, television, satellite dish, computer, bicycle, motorcycle and car	Lowest 20% of the sample on the assets index
5. Social participation	Community activities	Are you involved in community activities?	Does not participate
	Friendship	Do you have friends?	No friends
6.Psychological well-being	Depressed or anxious state	Are you depressed or feeling anxious?	Extremely anxious or depressed
	Feeling of happiness	Do you feel happy?	Never or almost never
7. Physical security	Maltreatment	Have you ever been mistreated?	Have been abused
	Sense of security	Do you feel safe?	Never, almost never or rarely

domain of deprivation is based on whether or not a person has paid employment. We considered only individuals between ages 18 and 65 so that children and elderly people were not considered poor in this dimension for the calculation of multidimensional poverty measures.

Our study included six indicators within the dimension of living conditions. Individuals who suffer from polluted indoor air because they use wood or coals to cook are considered poor on this dimension. Similarly, individuals who lack access to drinking water within their residence are also considered poor on the indicator of access to drinking water, and those without basic sanitation are considered poor, per the second target of MDG 7. For these three indicators, we refer to the official UNICEF definition for determining the threshold of acceptable hygiene. Our study also includes a measure of household occupancy rates within the dimension of living conditions (crowding space). The material well-being of a household is measured by an active indicator that includes a list of common property owned by the household.

Two indicators of social participation were included in our analysis. Participation in community activities assesses membership in a religious, cultural, social or sports organization. The ability to make friends is another important indicator of social inclusion. Scholars have demonstrated that persons with disabilities face prejudice and discrimination resulting in social exclusion (Mollica et al. 1999; World Bank 2009; Trani and Bakhshi 2011; Benoit et al. 2013). Stigmatized persons with disabilities face barriers to participation in the community and difficulties in connecting with other people (Meininger 2010). Two indicators of psychosocial well-being—feelings of anxiety or depression and feelings of happiness—were also included in the analysis. Furthermore, stigma and the resulting discrimination and social exclusion also impact self-esteem and result in psychological distress (Meyer, Schwartz, and Frost 2008). Both dimensions are important but are often neglected in poverty analysis (Alkire 2007).

Finally, two indicators of security and physical well-being were included in the analysis. Abuse and violence against persons with disabilities are depressingly prevalent in most countries (Branigan et al. 2001; Groce and Trasi 2004; Foster and Sandel 2010; Pestka and Wendt 2014). A sense of insecurity in one's neighborhood is considered an important element of vulnerability in the literature, and neighbors have often been identified among the perpetrators of violence (Wolbring 1994). The threshold (feeling that one lives in a somewhat or very dangerous environment) was determined by researchers and then tested in FGDs.

By taking into account a wide variety of dimensions of well-being, our study aims to identify differences in well-being between persons with disabilities and the rest of the population. We defined a threshold, d, determining multidimensional poverty: this poverty cut-off indicates the portion of weighted indicators in which a person has to be deprived to be considered multidimensionally poor. The cut-off is important: It determines which portion of the population is considered deprived and in need of urgent public policies to reduce poverty (Tsui 2002; Alkire and Foster 2011; Alkire et al. 2015). The cut-off was set at $d=40\%$ in Morocco and in Tunisia which leads to a rate of poverty of 29% and 15%, respectively. Although people interviewed were able to articulate a consensus view of the domains of difficulties they face in life, they did not reach a complete consensus defining the minimum set of deprivations that constitutes poverty. Results from FGDs and individual interviews suggest nevertheless that respondents in both countries identified same essential deprivations. Deprivation of social participation, education, health and material wealth together represent between 40% and 50% of all the deprivation indicators. In the present study, we show results for $d=40\%$. Sensitivity analysis demonstrated robustness of results to the choice of d value, particularly in terms of relative poverty between subgroups (data not shown).

3.5. Participatory Ranking Process

To assign weights to the different indicators within each dimension, we used a participatory ranking process based on the one described by Mitra et al. (2013). We organized additional FGDs in organizations of persons with disabilities in each country and presented each with the list of 17 indicators of poverty in seven well-being dimensions that had been identified via the literature search and prior FGDs in each country. Each group was instructed to discuss the importance that each of the 17 indicators held for persons with disabilities in that particular country. We asked groups to try to achieve consensus and to rank the 17 indicators in order of importance. Group members engaged in active debate and came to agreement in both countries.

We used two different methods to convert rankings into weights for the indicators within each dimension. We adapted the Alfares and Duffuaa (2008, 2009) method (AD method) and the De Krujik and Rutten (2007) method (DKR method) to account for the ranking by participants of indicators rather than dimensions. Within the equally weighted dimensions, we distributed the weight between indicators based on the rank assigned by participants and the number of indicators per dimension. Appendix 1 presents the results of the weighting using both methods. In both countries, the rank order of weighted indicators within dimensions was the same regardless of the method used.

3.6. Sensitivity Analysis of the Influence of Various Weight Structures on Multidimensional Poverty

To investigate if weights influenced multidimensional poverty estimates, we calculated the adjusted headcount ratio for three different weighting structures. Sen (1996) has argued that the relative value of dimensions of deprivation can be defined in various ways, primarily through public debate with people from relevant groups but also with local experts, through statistical analysis of available data, or by following the researcher's subjectivity (Sen 1996). Sen (1996) suggests that the choice should be made transparent and explicit, in order to allow space for discussion. However, regardless of weight structure considered, comparisons of relative multidimensional poverty between subgroups of population should remain unchanged.

Table 2 shows results for the adjusted headcount ratio for three different weighting structures and different poverty cut-offs *d*. Measure one is associated with the seven dimensions defined previously. Each dimension has an equal weight, as does each indicator within each dimension. Measures two and three transform rankings of indicators of deprivation by persons within the lived experience group into weights. Measure two converts individual ranking into weights for each individual who ranked the indicators and then calculates individual weights' average[1] (Alfares and Duffuaa 2008, 2009). Measure three establishes a collective ranking based on all individuals' ranking.[2] Results demonstrate that persons with disabilities are more deprived whatever the weighting structure. The relative structure of the adjusted headcount ratio M_0 for different subgroups remains unchanged when the weighting structure varies, demonstrating the robustness of our results. For the remaining parts of the paper, the analysis and results presented are based on the weighting structure of measure one.

3.7. Investigating Overlap of Deprivations: Correlations Between Indicators of Deprivation

We calculated Spearman rank correlation to look at associations between indicators of deprivation (see Appendix 2). Appendix 2 shows that poverty was better represented by

Table 2. Adjusted headcount ratio using for different weighting structures in Morocco and Tunisia

Morocco	Measure 1			Measure 2			Measure 3		
d (%)	All	PwDs	ND	All	PwDs	ND	All	PwDs	ND
10	0.180	0.214	0.145	0.169	0.204	0.133	0.167	0.202	0.132
20	0.168	0.206	0.130	0.157	0.195	0.119	0.152	0.189	0.115
30	0.133	0.174	0.091	0.117	0.159	0.073	0.116	0.159	0.072
40	0.091	0.130	0.051	0.076	0.115	0.035	0.075	0.115	0.034
50	0.057	0.092	0.022	0.043	0.073	0.012	0.043	0.073	0.013
60	0.021	0.037	0.004	0.018	0.032	0.003	0.017	0.031	0.003
70	0.006	0.011	0.001	0.005	0.01	0	0.005	0.011	0
80	0.001	0.002	0.000	0.001	0.002	0	0.001	0.002	0
Tunisia	Measure 1			Measure 2			Measure 3		
d (%)	All	PwDs	ND	All	PwDs	ND	All	PwDs	ND
10	0.138	0.171	0.108	0.121	0.157	0.089	0.127	0.161	0.097
20	0.124	0.159	0.093	0.096	0.136	0.061	0.099	0.14	0.063
30	0.073	0.107	0.043	0.06	0.098	0.027	0.061	0.099	0.028
40	0.043	0.07	0.019	0.028	0.048	0.01	0.031	0.052	0.013
50	0.021	0.037	0.007	0.009	0.017	0.002	0.009	0.017	0.002
60	0.005	0.009	0.001	0.001	0.002	0	0.001	0.003	NA

Note: Nobody is poor on more than eight indicators in Morocco and six indicators in Tunisia. PwDs, persons with disabilities; ND, non-disabled.

multiple dimensions than by a unique welfare indicator of poverty. We found a few correlations that were both significant and strong between indicators within a given dimension (for instance, not feeling happy and feeling depressed), but none between dimensions for both countries. In particular, individual-level basic capabilities—such as health, education, employment—and psychosocial dimensions were not correlated to household-level material well-being, justifying our choice of a multidimensional approach. There are a few exceptions: we found some associations (with a highest coefficient of 0.25 and 0.24, respectively, in Morocco and Tunisia) between indicators of material well-being and food security. Material poverty may result in poor diet as families struggle to secure enough food on a daily basis. We found a similar level of correlation between lack of education and social participation in both countries.

4. Results

4.1. Deprivation Rate by Indicator

The uncensored headcount ratio is reported in Figure 2. In both Morocco and Tunisia, deprivation is higher for a larger number of indicators for persons with disabilities compared to non-disabled people. In Tunisia, this is the case for 16 indicators out of 17. The gap is particularly high on all indicators of the dimensions of education, employment, social participation and psychological well-being. It is non-existent for indoor air pollution and close to null for quality of health care and type of lighting used. In Morocco, the uncensored headcount ratio is higher for persons with disabilities on 15 indicators. It is particularly high for indicators of the dimensions of employment, social participation, psychological well-being and physical safety. Access to clean water and type of lighting are slightly higher for non-disabled people. The gap in employment between both groups is strikingly similar in range and importance.

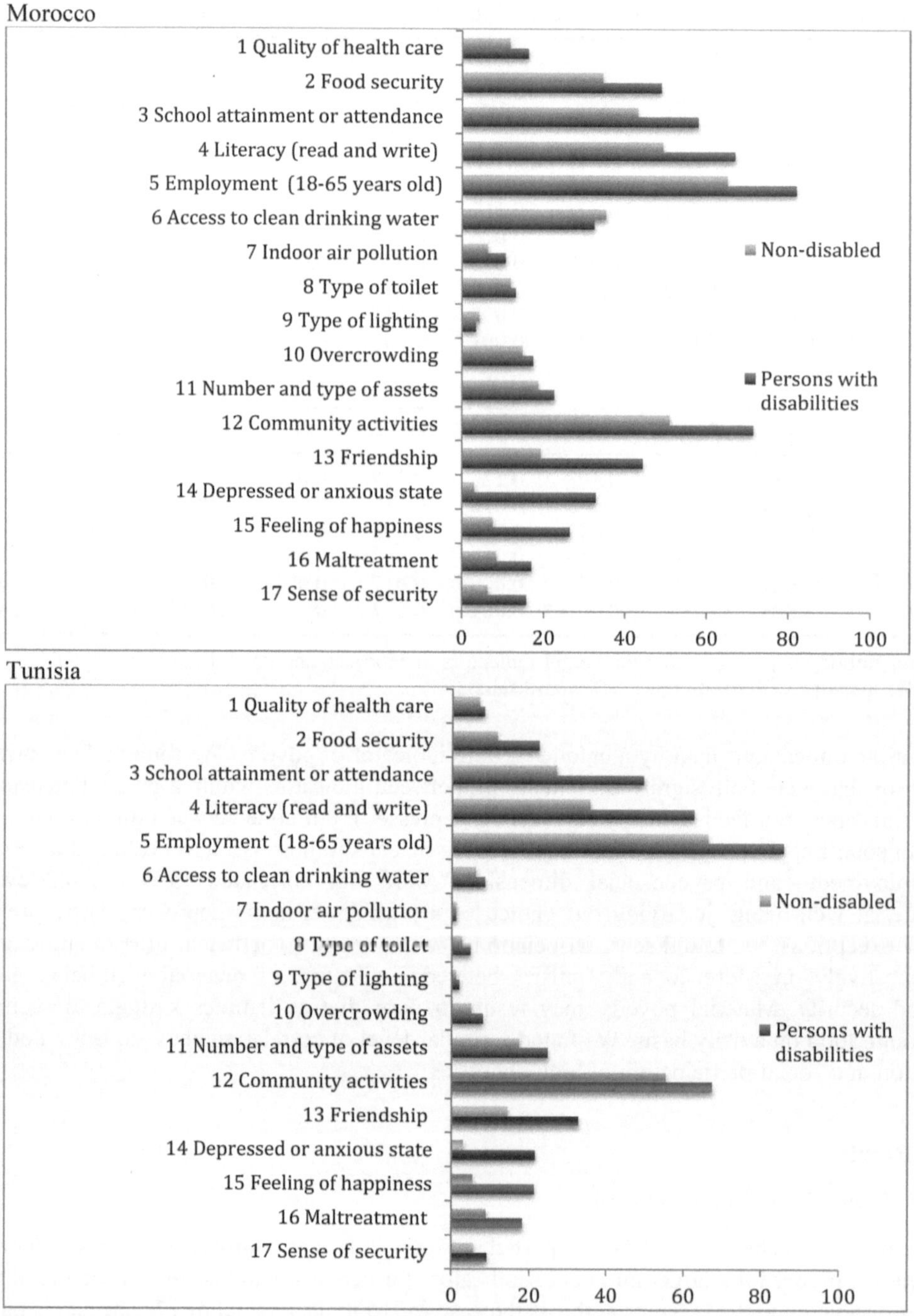

Figure 2. Deprivation rates by indicator and by disability status.

4.2. Multidimensional Poverty Results

Estimation of poverty headcount ratio H, intensity of poverty A and adjusted headcount ratio M_0 for various cut-offs d are presented in Table 3. Table 3 shows that nobody is deprived in all indicators, but more than half of Moroccans (50.4%) are deprived in 30% of the indicators and nearly two-thirds of Tunisians (64.9%) are deprived in 20% of

Table 3. Multidimensional poverty estimates for Morocco and Tunisia comparing persons with disabilities and non-disabled for various cut-off

	Morocco										Tunisia									
	All			Persons with disabilities			Non-disabled				All			Persons with disabilities			Non-disabled			
d	H	A	M_0	H	A	M_0	H	A	M_0	t value	H	A	M_0	H	A	M_0	H	A	M_0	t value
10	87.64	0.205	0.180	93.88	0.228	0.214	81.28	0.178	0.145	12.72	80.49	0.171	0.138	90.50	0.189	0.171	71.528	0.151	0.108	11.88
20	74.53	0.225	0.168	84.33	0.244	0.206	64.54	0.201	0.130	12.22	64.93	0.191	0.124	77.71	0.205	0.159	53.472	0.173	0.093	11.15
30	50.41	0.264	0.133	62.54	0.278	0.174	38.05	0.240	0.091	11.20	29.85	0.245	0.073	42.44	0.253	0.107	18.576	0.229	0.043	9.61
40	29.62	0.306	0.091	41.04	0.316	0.130	17.96	0.282	0.051	10.49	15.02	0.286	0.043	24.03	0.289	0.070	6.944	0.276	0.019	8.26
50	16.73	0.343	0.057	26.42	0.348	0.092	6.85	0.324	0.022	10.20	6.50	0.327	0.021	11.24	0.329	0.037	2.257	0.322	0.007	6.13
60	5.20	0.399	0.021	9.25	0.399	0.037	1.07	0.394	0.004	6.82	1.19	0.386	0.005	2.33	0.386	0.009	0.174	0.378	0.001	3.30
70	1.36	0.444	0.006	2.54	0.446	0.011	0.15	0.420	0.001	3.79	0	NA	NA	0	NA	NA	0	NA	NA	NA
80	0.23	0.500	0.001	0.45	0.500	0.002	0.00	NA	0.000	1.72	0	NA	NA	0	NA	NA	0	NA	NA	NA

Note: Nobody is deprived on more than 80% of dimensions in Morocco and 60% of dimensions in Tunisia. t-test value all significant at 0.001.

indicators. Furthermore, findings show that whatever the cut-off d, the adjusted headcount ratio is higher in Morocco than in Tunisia. In both countries, the adjusted headcount ratio is significantly higher ($p < .01$) for persons with disabilities compared to non-disabled persons. The difference in the adjusted headcount ratio across disability status is higher in Morocco than in Tunisia whatever the cut-off d.

Table 4 compares multidimensional poverty estimates for disability status as well as for various subgroups of interest. Analysis yields important variations according to gender, age, residence, disability status and type. First, in both countries, a higher headcount ratio H is observed for persons with disabilities than for non-disabled people: 36.7% in Morocco compared to 25.5%, and 24% compared to 7% in Tunisia. Other authors found similar patterns (Mitra, Posarac, and Vick 2013; Trani and Cannings 2013; Trani, Biggeri, and Mauro 2013). Second, average deprivation share A and adjusted headcount ratio M_0 are also higher for persons with disabilities. The difference in adjusted headcount ratio is explained by a significant gap in both headcount ratio and average deprivation share in Morocco. In Tunisia, the gap in A is less significant than the difference in H explaining most of the difference in multidimensional poverty between disabled and non-disabled people. In fact, the average poor person with disabilities is deprived in 41% and 49.2% of the weighted indicators, respectively, compared to 18% and 47% for non-disabled people, respectively, in Morocco and Tunisia. Third, multidimensional poverty is found to be higher in women and girls with disabilities in both countries. Trani and Cannings (2013) and Trani, Biggeri, and Mauro (2013) also found, respectively, in Darfur and Afghanistan, that girls with disabilities compared to boys had higher adjusted multidimensional poverty headcounts. Fourth, adjusted headcount ratio is higher for working-age people with disabilities than for children and elderly adults with disabilities. Mitra et al. (2013) also found that working-age adults with disabilities were more likely to be poor than non-disabled people. This was also the case in 12 out of 15 countries studied for elderly people (above 60). Fifth, persons with multiple disabilities in both countries were found to be multidimensionally poorer than persons with any single type of disability. Trani and Cannings (2013) in Darfur and Mitra et al. (2013) in 12 countries also found higher adjusted headcounts for persons with multiple disabilities compared to persons with a single disability. Persons with intellectual or mental disability in Tunisia and persons with moderate severity of disability in Morocco rank second for adjusted headcount ratio. Conversely, Trani and Cannings (2013) found that children with intellectual disabilities in Darfur were the least multidimensionally poor among children with disabilities. In both countries, people with moderate degree of any type of disability are poorer than people with severe physical or sensory disability.

Table 5 presents the poverty headcount in each dimension—that is, the share of the poor who are deprived in each dimension—by disability status, gender, age group, place of residence, disability type and severity. Whatever the indicator, H is higher for persons with disabilities compared to non-disabled people. The gap is particularly high in the dimensions of health, education, material well-being, social participation and psychological well-being in both countries, as well as for physical safety only in Morocco. The level of H is higher for women than for men with disabilities in 11 indicators out of 17 in both countries. The gap is the highest for education in both countries. Social participation represents a relatively large gap in H in both countries. The gap is also high for employment in Morocco. Poverty headcount is higher for persons with disabilities living in rural areas than for those living in urban areas in both countries: this is the case for 12 indicators in Morocco and 11 in Tunisia. The gap is particularly significant for access to water and sanitation in both countries. In Morocco, we observe a relatively large gap for food security, employment, education, social participation and depression or anxiety. In Tunisia, there is a large

Table 4. Multidimensional poverty estimates for Morocco and Tunisia by disability status, gender, age group, place of residence and type of disability

Morocco $d = 40\%$	H	A	M_0
All	31.17	0.296	0.154
Disability status			
Disabled	36.7	0.41	0.22
Non-disabled	25.53	0.18	0.086
Gender			
Men disabled	34.08	0.376	0.2
Men non-disabled	19.68	0.072	0.033
Women disabled	39.45	0.446	0.242
Women non-disabled	31.54	0.29	0.14
Age group			
Disabled below 18	25.72	0.136	0.072
Non-disabled below 18	12.73	0.04	0.018
Disabled 18–65	38.88	0.486	0.266
Non-disabled 18–65	24.79	0.11	0.053
Disabled over 65	37.69	0.43	0.23
Non-disabled over 65	27.73	0.218	0.105
Residence			
Rabat disabled	35.1	0.366	0.191
Rabat non-disabled	24.55	0.177	0.085
Chaouia disabled	38.08	0.449	0.246
Chaouia non-disabled	26.34	0.182	0.087
Type and degree of disability			
Non-disabled	25.53	0.18	0.086
Moderate degree of disability	35.09	0.406	0.214
High degree physical	34.57	0.35	0.187
High degree sensory	34	0.34	0.181
High degree intellectual and mental	34.21	0.382	0.208
High degree multiple disability	39.96	0.48	0.259

Tunisia $d = 40\%$	H	A	M_0
All	15.01	0.486	0.073
Disability status			
Disabled	24.03	0.492	0.118
Non-disabled	6.94	0.47	0.033
Gender			
Men disabled	22.47	0.479	0.108
Men non-disabled	1.98	0.462	0.009
Women disabled	25.26	0.501	0.127
Women non-disabled	10.84	0.471	0.051
Age group			
Disabled below 18	4.76	0.452	0.022
Non-disabled below 18	0	NA	0
Disabled 18–65	38.43	0.497	0.191
Non-disabled 18–65	9.61	0.471	0.045
Disabled over 65	10.96	0.472	0.052
Non-disabled over 65	0.78	0.429	0.003
Residence			
Tunis disabled	24.32	0.493	0.12
Tunis non-disabled	4.38	0.478	0.021
Béja disabled	23.66	0.49	0.116
Béja non-disabled	10.16	0.465	0.047

(*Continued*)

Table 4. Continued

Morocco $d = 40\%$	H	A	M_0
Type and degree of disability			
Non-disabled	6.94	0.47	0.033
Moderate degree of disability	18.67	0.509	0.095
High degree physical	17.2	0.481	0.083
High degree sensory	9.09	0.486	0.044
High degree intellectual and mental	32.14	0.471	0.151
High degree multiple disability	34.68	0.5	0.173

difference in the poverty headcount between rural and urban persons with disabilities on the indicator for material wealth. In both countries, H is higher for adults with disabilities, particularly for education, employment and social participation and to a lesser extent for food security and psychological well-being. The highest level of H is also observed in both countries for multiple disabilities followed by intellectual and mental and physical or moderate disabilities. People with multiple disabilities show the highest headcount ratio on ten and eight indicators in Morocco and Tunisia, respectively.

Finally, we show the percent contribution of each dimension to the overall adjusted headcount ratio M_0 in Appendix 3 for the chosen cut-offs. In both countries, in both urban and rural areas, for both male and female adults, whatever the disability status and type, deprivation in employment is the leading contributor to poverty. This finding differs from Mitra et al. (2013) who found that non-health per capita expenditure was the major contributor to M_0 followed by education and then employment in almost all countries. The contribution of employment is even higher for non-disabled people in our study. Overall, contributions to M_0 are similar whatever the disability status. Yet, we observe a relative higher contribution of indicators of psychological well-being for persons with disabilities, whatever the disability type. In both countries, the second weighted indicator's contribution is participation in community activities for persons with disabilities compared to literacy for persons without disabilities. Participation in community activities is third for persons without disabilities while it is literacy for persons with disabilities.

The contributions from indicators of psychological well-being and physical safety are substantially higher for persons with disabilities in both countries; this is true for both men and women. In both countries, mistreatment contributes more to multidimensional poverty for men, regardless of disability. In Tunisia, depression/anxiety is an important contributor to multidimensional poverty for both persons with disabilities and non-disabled men. For women in Tunisia and for men and women in Morocco, this contribution is small for those without disabilities compared to those with disabilities. All six indicators of deprivation of living conditions have low contributions to overall poverty in both countries, in both rural and urban areas and in both households with and without persons with disabilities. This reflects the level of economic development of the two countries and the achievement of major development milestones for the overall population. On a similar note, it is striking that deprivation of quality of health care contributes less than 5% to overall poverty and that its contribution to poverty is lower among persons with disabilities than among non-disabled people. Yet, the difference is limited and can again be justified by the relative importance of other indicators to the adjusted headcount ratio M_0.

Table 5. Headcount ratio H per dimension for $d = 40\%$

Morocco	Quality of health care	Food security	School attainment/ attendance	Literacy (read and write)	Non-employment (18–65)	Access to clean drinking water	Indoor air pollution	Type of toilet	Type of lighting	Over-crowded space	Number and type of assets	Community activities	Friendship	Depressed/ anxious state	Feeling of happiness	Maltreat-ment	Sense of security
All	6.98	20.15	22.08	24.66	23.21	12.3	4.9	6.34	2.04	6.12	9.49	24.19	19.82	12.39	11.84	6.33	7.39
Disability status																	
Cases	10	28.74	28.81	32.99	30.6	16.62	7.31	8.55	2.24	8.4	13.14	34.33	29.4	22.87	20.3	10.15	12.11
Control	4.06	11.42	15.22	16.16	15.68	7.91	2.44	4.11	1.83	3.81	5.8	13.85	10.05	1.68	3.2	2.44	2.59
Gender																	
Men disabled	9.32	26.61	21.28	25.66	27.11	16.72	7.29	7.04	2.34	8.5	10.29	32.07	26.53	21.05	21.87	12.24	12.57
Men non-disabled	2.74	5.11	5.71	5.72	4.8	3.6	0.9	2.7	0.9	1.8	2.7	5.41	3	0.9	1.5	1.8	0.9
Women disabled	10.68	30.98	36.7	40.67	34.25	16.51	7.34	10.12	2.14	8.28	16.15	36.7	32.42	24.77	18.65	7.95	11.62
Women non-disabled	5.43	17.9	25	26.85	26.85	12.35	4.01	5.56	2.78	5.88	9.01	22.53	17.28	2.48	4.95	3.09	4.32
Age group																	
Cases below 18	4.76	9.09	7.58	12.12	0	7.58	6.06	1.52	0	6.06	7.58	10.61	10.61	7.58	12.12	9.09	7.58
Controls below 18	2.7	4	1.33	2.67	0	4	0	3	0	1	0	4	4	1	0	2.67	0
Cases 18–65	13	31.19	26.61	33.94	44.04	20.18	9.17	11.11	1.85	9.26	11.21	42.2	33.03	27.52	26.61	14.68	16.51
Controls 18–65	2.75	4.59	8.26	8.26	10.09	5.5	0.92	3.67	0.92	1.83	2.75	11.01	9.17	0	0.92	1	2.75
Cases over 65	10.07	30.83	32.12	35.56	31.72	17.04	7.07	8.92	2.63	8.52	14.31	35.76	31.11	23.89	20	9.29	11.74
Controls over 65	4.59	14.16	19.03	20.13	19.45	9.09	3.17	4.44	2.33	4.66	7.43	16.07	11.21	2.12	4.24	2.75	2.96
Residence																	
Rabat cases	9.97	23.95	22.65	28.48	26.21	5.83	9.71	1.96	1.29	6.19	13.25	31.39	25.89	19.48	18.45	8.74	14.24
Rabat controls	2.72	10.37	14.72	15.72	16.72	2.68	4.01	0.67	1	2.35	4.71	15.38	11.71	1.35	4.03	1.34	3.01

(Continued)

Table 5. Continued

Morocco	Quality of health care	Food security	School attainment/ attendance	Literacy (read and write)	Non-employment (18–65)	Access to clean drinking water	Indoor air pollution	Type of toilet	Type of lighting	Over-crowded space	Number and type of assets	Community activities	Friendship	Depressed/ anxious state	Feeling of happiness	Maltreat-ment	Sense of security
Chaouia cases	10.03	32.87	34.07	36.84	34.35	25.91	5.26	14.13	3.06	10.28	13.06	36.84	32.41	25.76	21.88	11.36	10.28
Chaouia controls	5.19	12.29	15.64	16.53	14.8	12.29	1.12	6.98	2.51	5.03	6.7	12.57	8.66	1.96	2.51	3.35	2.23
Type of disability																	
Non-disabled	4.06	11.42	15.22	16.16	15.68	7.91	2.44	4.11	1.83	3.81	5.8	13.85	10.05	1.68	3.2	2.44	2.59
Moderate disability	10.94	31.88	26.09	30.43	31.88	1.59	7.25	11.59	1.45	4.35	17.65	33.33	21.74	23.19	11.59	15.94	13.04
Physical	5.16	29.45	27.61	31.9	26.99	16.67	4.29	8.02	4.32	9.32	14.38	26.99	23.31	17.18	14.72	6.13	6.13
Sensory	8.89	21.88	13.4	21.65	26.8	12.37	8.25	8.25	3.09	5.15	12.37	27.84	26.8	19.59	18.56	10.31	15.46
Intellectual and mental	12.9	32.35	23.53	30.88	29.41	14.93	5.88	10.29	0	7.35	16.18	27.94	26.47	25	19.12	5.88	11.76
Multiple	12.45	29.04	37	38.83	34.07	19.78	9.16	7.75	1.47	10.29	10.78	42.86	36.63	26.84	26.74	12.09	14.34
Tunisia																	
All	2.47	7.23	9.07	12.18	12.36	.83	0.27	1.37	0.27	2.66	5.86	13.37	9.34	6.14	6.32	4.67	2.66
Disability status																	
Cases	0	11.24	13.95	18.6	18.6	2.33	0.58	1.94	0.39	4.65	9.11	21.71	15.89	11.82	12.6	8.33	4.65
Controls	1.91	3.65	4.69	6.42	6.77	1.39	0	0.87	0.17	0.87	2.95	5.9	3.47	1.04	0.69	1.39	0.87
Gender																	
Men disabled	3.52	10.13	8.81	15.42	19.38	3.08	0	1.32	0	6.17	8.81	19.82	12.78	10.57	12.78	8.37	3.08
Men non-disabled	1.58	0.79	0.79	1.19	1.58	0	0	0	0	0	0.4	1.58	1.19	0.79	0.79	0.4	0.4
Women disabled	2.77	12.11	17.99	21.11	17.99	1.73	1.04	2.42	0.69	3.46	9.34	23.18	18.34	12.8	12.46	8.3	5.88
Women non-disabled	2.17	5.88	7.74	10.53	10.84	2.48	0	1.55	0.31	1.55	4.95	9.29	5.26	1.24	0.62	2.17	1.24
Age group																	
Cases below 18	2.38	0	4.76	4.76	0	0	0	0	0	2.38	2.38	4.76	2.38	2.38	4.76	2.38	0

Controls below 18	0	0	0	0	0	0	0	0	0	0	0	0	0	0	0	0	0
Cases 18–65	4.71	17.65	18.04	27.45	37.65	3.92	0.39	1.57	0.39	7.45	13.73	34.9	23.92	16.86	17.65	14.9	7.06
Controls 18–65	2.46	5.17	6.4	8.87	9.61	1.97	0	1.23	0.25	1.23	4.19	8.13	4.68	1.48	0.99	1.72	1.23
Cases over 65	1.37	5.94	10.96	10.96	0	0.91	0.91	2.74	0.46	1.83	5.02	9.59	9.13	7.76	8.22	1.83	2.74
Controls over 65	0.78	0	0.78	0.78	0	0	0	0	0	0	0	0.78	0.78	0	0	0.78	0
Residence																	
Tunis cases	2.74	13.01	13.36	18.15	18.84	0	0	0.34	0.34	2.4	6.51	22.95	15.07	14.04	14.38	7.88	5.48
Tunis controls	0.94	3.44	1.88	3.75	4.38	0.31	0	0	0.31	0	0.94	4.06	2.81	0.94	0.63	0.94	0.63
Béja cases	3.57	8.93	14.73	19.2	18.3	5.36	1.34	4.02	0.45	7.59	12.5	20.09	16.96	8.93	10.27	8.93	3.57
Béja controls	3.13	3.91	8.2	9.77	9.77	2.73	0	1.95	0	1.95	5.47	8.2	4.3	1.17	0.78	1.95	1.17
Type of disability																	
Non-disabled	1.91	3.65	4.69	6.42	6.77	1.39	0	0.87	0.17	0.87	2.95	5.9	3.47	1.04	0.69	1.39	0.87
Moderate disability	2.67	12	8	9.33	17.33	0	1.33	2.67	1.33	4	9.33	16	12	8	9.33	10.67	4
Physical	1.91	10.19	8.28	14.01	12.74	1.27	0.64	2.55	0	5.73	10.19	15.92	6.37	11.46	8.28	5.1	1.91
Sensory	1.82	3.64	9.09	9.09	7.27	3.64	0	0	0	1.82	0	7.27	7.27	1.82	3.64	1.82	0
Intellectual and mental	3.57	16.07	8.93	21.43	26.79	5.36	1.79	1.79	0	0	16.07	28.57	17.86	10.71	17.86	14.29	10.71
Multiple	4.62	12.72	24.86	28.9	25.43	2.89	0	1.73	0.58	6.36	8.67	31.79	28.32	17.34	19.08	10.4	6.94

5. Concluding Remarks

The present paper provides estimates of multidimensional poverty in Morocco and Tunisia comparing the situation of persons with and without disabilities using three measures of multidimensional poverty, (i) the headcount ratio H, (ii) the average share of deprivations A and (iii) M_0, the adjusted headcount ratio following Alkire and Foster (2011). Findings were tested for robustness of estimates by changing the dimensions' weighting structure. Comparing multidimensional poverty estimates across different weighting structures, the relative position of the disabled and non-disabled did not change, demonstrating stability of the findings. This study highlights three important conclusions linked to poverty that could guide public policy and improve circumstances of persons with disabilities in both countries within a social justice perspective.

First, overall results indicate that persons with disabilities face higher levels and intensity of multidimensional poverty in both Morocco and Tunisia, not just in the field of employment. This reflects the "double handicap" that persons with disabilities face (Sen 1992, 2009). Disability is associated with a lower capacity to earn an income because of inadequate participation in the workforce; Sen calls this the "earning handicap." In fact, findings demonstrate that the major contributor to multidimensional poverty in both countries is non-employment and reflects current economic challenges. Non-employment is widespread, but the situation is worse for persons with disabilities, particularly women. High rates of unemployment in Morocco and Tunisia generally make it more challenging for policy-makers to specifically promote employment of persons with disabilities. Yet, organizations of persons with disabilities and wider civil society should advocate for better participation in the workforce not through the mere creation of employment opportunities but by fighting the discrimination and stigma found to be very high in both countries (Bakhshi et al. 2014a, b).

Sen (1992, 2009) also argues that disability is associated with a "conversion handicap" linked to the extra costs incurred by disability. In order to cope with impairment and live a good life, persons with disabilities need more access to existing resources (Braithwaite and Mont 2009). The current economic situation in Morocco and Tunisia makes the implementation of social policy difficult. Even though basic livelihood conditions such as water, sanitation and decent housing have been improved during the development efforts carried out in both countries, levels of deprivation of material well-being and food security for persons with disabilities, particularly in rural areas, remain high.

Second, multidimensional poverty is higher for certain subgroups. For example, poverty is greater for both women with and without disability compared to men. In other words, there are more women and men with disabilities who are multidimensionally poor in both countries, but among the deprived, the intensity of poverty is higher for women, particularly those with disabilities. Such findings illustrate the so-called "double burden" of being disabled and being a woman (World Health Organization and World Bank 2011). Literature shows that women with disabilities are more likely than any other group to be deprived of essential capabilities in LMICs (Groce 1997). Women with disabilities in Morocco and Tunisia are particularly deprived of education compared to men with disabilities. We observe similar findings for other subgroups, such as persons living in rural areas.

Third, several dimensions of deprivation reflect phenomena of prejudice and stigma toward persons with disabilities. Both indicators of social participation show higher poverty for persons with disabilities. These findings highlight that stigma is a major issue: discriminatory attitudes resulting from prejudice lead to persons with disabilities being viewed as second-class citizens who are entitled to collective assistance, but not entitled to the same opportunities and freedom to choose to be and to do what they value (Sen 1999). This constitutes an important source of mental distress for persons with disabilities living in countries, as they are viewed primarily as recipients of charity. Consequently, persons with disabilities are highly deprived of psychological well-being as measured by their state of anxiety and depression and their feeling of unhappiness. Barriers to social participation are often invisible (prejudice) or linked to the environment and infrastructure (accessibility issues) as shown in the literature on disability in LMICs (Maart et al. 2007; de Klerk 2008; Mirza et al. 2009; Isaac, Dharma Raja, and Ravanan 2010). Widespread and persistent negative attitudes and discrimination lead to frustration and low self-esteem (Mashiach-Eizenberg et al. 2013; Nario-Redmond, Noel, and Fern 2013).

Our study contributes to a better understanding of the material and emotional needs of persons with disabilities and highlights deficiencies in their "well-being freedom" and poverty reduction in general (Drydyk 2012). The findings shed light on deep-rooted injustice for persons with disabilities, particularly girls and women, rural residents, and those with intellectual, mental or multiple disabilities. In both countries, the disproportionate share of poverty is borne by persons with disabilities and women, illustrating a lack of equal opportunity and freedom in several areas. It is imperative to identify the capabilities in which persons with disabilities may be deprived, as this helps to better decipher "the barriers societies have erected against full justice" (Nussbaum 2003, 33). By showing deprivation of basic capabilities and functionings, our findings demonstrate inequality of opportunities for persons with disabilities in both Moroccan and Tunisian societies. These findings constitute a social justice agenda for civil society in general and particularly organizations of persons with disabilities: a valuable basis to lobby for more just policies and hold policy-makers accountable to making tangible progress. A central implication of our findings is the need to address stigma and discrimination as a priority: civil society organizations should take the lead to promote awareness of social and emotional well-being of persons with disabilities. Literature has demonstrated that the poor and vulnerable, those marginalized in a given society, can collectively exert agency to promote positive change for themselves and for the group (Ibrahim 2006; Dubois et al. 2008; Dubois and Trani 2009). Localized and specific interventions at the community level, where persons with disabilities live, have been shown to be more effective to promote inclusion, increase self-esteem, and can complement national sensitization campaigns (Ntshangase, Mdikana, and Cronk 2008; Corrigan and Fong 2014).

Finally, our findings have important implications for both countries in terms of public policies aiming at improving economic and social inclusion of persons with disabilities. Public policies relying solely on a social approach are ineffective to change the status quo. Interventions such as awareness, advocacy and campaigns to fight stigma (specifically toward women and persons with multiple disabilities) are necessary to be placed alongside policies promoting equal opportunities and equal access, particularly to the labor market. In Morocco and Tunisia, better implementation and enforcement of existing legislation are needed to promote equality of capabilities for persons with disabilities.

Notes

1. The following equation is used to change of individual rankings into individual weights:$w_{ij} = 100 - S_n(r_{ij} - 1)$ With w_{ij} weight of the dimension for the individual , r_{ij} represents the ranking of dimension j for the individual i, n is the overall number of individuals involved in the ranking process. S_n is a parameter given by the following formula: $S_n = 3.195 + \frac{37.758}{n}$

2. The weight of dimension j is determined by the following equation: $w_j = \dfrac{1 + d - r_j}{1 + d - \sum_{j-1}^{d} r_j}$

   With d the number of dimensions and r_j the classification of dimension j with a value of 1 if this is the most important dimension, 2 if it is the second most important and so on.

Disclosure statement

No potential conflict of interest was reported by the authors.

References

Alfares, H. K., and S. O. Duffuaa. 2008. "Determining Aggregate Criteria Weights from Criteria Rankings By a Group of Decision Makers." *International Journal of Information Technology and Decision Making* 7 (4): 769–781.

Alfares, H. K., and S. O. Duffuaa. 2009. "Assigning Cardinal Weights in Multi-Criteria Decision Making Based on Ordinal Ranking." *Journal of Multi-Criteria Decision Analysis*, 15 (5–6): 125–133.

Alkire, S. 2002. "Dimensions of Human Development." *World Development* 30 (2): 181–205.

Alkire, S. 2007. "The Missing Dimensions of Poverty Data: Introduction to the Special Issue." *Oxford Development Studies* 35 (4): 347–359.

Alkire, S. 2008. "Choosing Dimensions: The Capability Approach and Multidimensional Poverty." In *Many Dimensions of Poverty*, edited by N. Kakwani and J. Silber, 89–119. New York: Palgrave Macmillan.

Alkire, Sabina, and James Foster. 2011. "Counting and Multidimensional Poverty Measurement." *Journal of Public Economics* 95 (7–8): 476–487.

Alkire, Sabina, James Foster, Suman Seth, Maria Emma Santos, Jose Manuel Roche, and Paola Ballon. 2015. "Multidimensional Poverty Measurement and Analysis: Chapter 6–Normative Choices in Measurement Design." In *Multidimensional Poverty Measurement and Analysis*, edited by Sabina Alkire, James Foster, Suman Seth, Maria Emma Santos, Jose Manuel Roche, and Paola Ballon, 241–283. Oxford: Oxford University Press.

Alkire, S., and M. E. Santos. 2014. "Measuring Acute Poverty in the Developing World: Robustness and Scope of the Multidimensional Poverty Index." *World Development* 59: 251–274.

Bakhshi, P., F. Gall, D. Lopez, and J. F. Trani. 2014a. "Le handicap dans les politiques publiques marocaines face au creusement des inégalités et à l'appauvrissement des familles avec des ayants droit handicapés." In *Collection Recherche et Études*, 130. Rabat: Handicap International.

Bakhshi, P., F. Gall, D. Lopez, and J. F. Trani. 2014b. *Le handicap dans les politiques publiques tunisiennes face au creusement des inégalités et à l'appauvrissement des familles avec des ayants droit en situation de handicap*. Tunis: Handicap International, 134.

Barclay, L. 2012. "Natural Deficiency or Social Oppression? The Capabilities Approach to Justice for People with Disabilities." *Journal of Moral Philosophy* 9 (4): 500–520.

Benoit, C., M. Jansson, M. Jansenberger, and R. Phillips. 2013. "Disability Stigmatization as a Barrier to Employment Equity for Legally-blind Canadians." *Disability and Society* 28 (7): 970–983.

Bourguignon, F., and S. Chakravarty. 2003. "The Measurement of Multidimensional Poverty." *Journal of Economic Inequality* 1: 25–49.

Braithwaite, J., and D. Mont. 2009. "Disability and Poverty: A Survey of World Bank Poverty Assessments and Implications." *ALTER European Journal of Disability Research* 3 (3): 219–232.

Branigan, M., D. E. Stewart, G. S. Tardif, and A. Veltman. 2001. "Perceptions of Primary Healthcare Services Among Persons with Physical Disabilities—Part 2: Quality Issues." *Medscape General Medicine* 3 (2): 19.

Chapireau, F. 2002. "La nouvelle classification de l'OMS : Classification internationale du fonctionnement, du handicap et de la santé." *Annales Médico-psychologiques* 160: 242–246.

Chiappero-Martinetti, E. 2000. "A multidimensional Assessment of Well-Being based on SEN's Functioning Approach." *Societa italiana di Economia Pubblica,* Working paper, *Rivista Internazionale di Scienze Sociali* 2.

Chiappero-Martinetti, E., and S. Moroni. 2007. "An Analytical Framework for Conceptualizing Poverty and Re-Examining the Capability Approach." *Journal of Socio-Economics* 36 (3): 360–375.

Corrigan, P. W., and M. W. M. Fong. 2014. "Competing Perspectives on Erasing the Stigma of Illness: What Says the Dodo Bird?" *Social Science and Medicine* 103: 110–117.

De Kruijk, H., and M. Rutten. 2007. "Weighting Dimensions of Poverty Based on Peoples Priorities: Constructing a Composite Poverty Index for the Maldives." Q-squared working paper, 35.

Deutsch, J., and J. G. Silber. 2005. "Measuring Multidimensional Poverty: An Empirical Comparison of Various Approaches." *Review of Income and Wealth* 51: 145–174.

Drydyk, J. 2012. "A Capability Approach to Justice as a Virtue." *Ethical Theory and Moral Practice* 15 (1): 23–38.

Dubois, J. L., A. S. Brouillet, P. Bakhshi, and C. Duray-Soundron, eds. 2008. "Repenser l'action collective. Une approche par les capabilites." In *Ethique ecoonomique*, edited by F.-R. Mahieu, 280. Paris: L'Harmattan.

Dubois, J. L., and J. F. Trani. 2009. "Extending the Capability Paradigm to Address the Complexity of Disability." *ALTER European Journal of Disability Research* 3 (3): 192–218.

Eide, A. H., and M. Loeb. 2006. *Living Conditions among People with Activity Limitations in Zambia: A National Representative Study.* Oslo: SINTEF Health Research.

Erb, S., and B. Harris-White. 2001. "The Economic Impact and Developmental Implications of Disability and Incapacity in Adulthood in a Village Study from S. India" Paper presented Welfare, demography and development Workshop, Downing College, Cambridge, September 11–12.

Filmer, D. 2008. "Disability, Poverty and Schooling in Developing Countries: Results from 14 Household Surveys." *The World Bank Economic Review* 22: 141–163.

Foster, K., and M. Sandel. 2010. "Abuse of Women with Disabilities: Toward an Empowerment Perspective." *Sexuality and Disability* 28 (3): 177–186.

Freire, P. 1970. *Pedagogy of the Oppressed.* New York, NY: Continuum.

Gartrell, Alexandra. 2010. ""A Frog in a Well": The Exclusion of Disabled People from Work in Cambodia." *Disability and Society* 25 (3): 289–301. http://www.informaworld.com/openurl?genre=article&id=doi:10.1080/09687591003701207.

Groce, Nora E. 1997. "Women with Disabilities in the Developing World." *Journal of Disability Policy Studies* 8 (1–2): 177–193.

Groce, N., and R. Trasi. 2004. "Rape of Individuals with Disability: AIDS and the Folk Belief of "Virgin Cleansing"." *The Lancet* 363: 1663–1664.

Grut, L., and B. Ingstad. 2006. *This is My Life: Living with a Disability in Yemen—A Qualitative Study.* Oslo: SINTEF Health Research. Accessed August 14, 2015. http://siteresources.worldbank.org/DISABILITY/Resources/Regions/ Africa/LCYemen.pdf.

Hamonet, C., and T. Magalhaes. 2003. "La Notion de Handicap." *Annales de Réadaption Médicale et Physique* 46: 521–524.

Ibrahim, S. S. 2006. "From Individual to Collective Capabilities: The Capability Approach as a Conceptual Framework for Self-help." *Journal of Human Development* 7 (3): 397–416.

Ingstad, B., and L. Grut. 2007. *See Me and Do not Forget me: People with Disabilities in Kenya.* Oslo: SINTEF Health Research. Accessed September 12, 2015. http://hpod.pmhclients.com/pdf/SeemeKenya2.pdf.

Isaac, Rebecca, B. William Dharma Raja, and M. P. Ravanan. 2010. "Integrating People with Disabilities: Their Right—Our Responsibility." *Disability and Society* 25 (5): 627–630. URL: http://www.informaworld.com/openurl?genre=article&id=doi:10.1080/09687599.2010.489314.

de Klerk, Ton. 2008. "Funding for Self-employment of People with Disabilities. Grants, Loans, Revolving Funds or Linkage with Microfinance Programmes." *Leprosy Review* 79 (1): 92–109.

Maart, S., A. H. Eide, J. Jelsma, M. E. Loeb, and M. Ka Toni. 2007. "Environmental Barriers Experienced by Urban and Rural Disabled People in South Africa." *Disability and Society* 22 (4): 357–369. http://www.informaworld.com/openurl?genre=article&id=doi:10.1080/09687590701337678.

Mashiach-Eizenberg, M., I. Hasson-Ohayon, P. T. Yanos, P. H. Lysaker, and D. Roe. 2013. "Internalized Stigma and Quality of Life among Persons with Severe Mental Illness: The Mediating Roles of Self-esteem and Hope." *Psychiatry Research* 208 (1): 15–20.

Meininger, H. P. 2010. "Connecting Stories: A Narrative Approach of Social Inclusion of Persons with Intellectual Disability." *Alter* 4 (3): 190–202. doi:10.1016/j.alter.2010.04.001.

Meyer, Ilan H., Sharon Schwartz, and David M. Frost. 2008. "Social Patterning of Stress and Coping: Does Disadvantaged Social Statuses Confer more Stress and Fewer Coping Resources?" *Social Science & Medicine* 67 (3): 368–379. doi:10.1016/j.socscimed.2008.03.012.

Mirza, I., A. Tareen, L. L. Davidson, and A. Rahman. 2009. "Community Management of Intellectual Disabilities in Pakistan: A Mixed Methods Study." *Journal of Intellectual Disability Research* 53 (6): 559–570.

Mitra, S. 2006. "The Capability Approach and Disability." *Journal of Disability Policy Studies* 16 (4): 236–247.

Mitra, S., K. Jones, B. Vick, D. Brown, E. McGinn, and M. J. Alexander. 2013. "Implementing a Multidimensional Poverty Measure Using Mixed Methods and a Participatory Framework." *Social Indicators Research* 110 (3): 1061–1081.

Mitra, S., A. Posarac, and B. Vick. 2013. "Disability and Poverty in Developing Countries: A Multidimensional Study." *World Development* 41 (1): 1–18.

Mitra, S., and U. Sambamoorthi. 2008. "Disability and the Rural Labor Market in India: Evidence for Males in Tamil Nadu." *World Development* 36 (5): 934–952.

Mitra, S., and U. Sambamoorthi. 2009. "Wage Differential by Disability Status in an Agrarian Labor Market in India." *Applied Economics Letters* 16 (14): 1393–1398.

Mizunoya, S., and S. Mitra. 2013. "Is There a Disability Gap in Employment Rates in Developing Countries?" *World Development* 42 (1): 28–43.

Mollica, R. F, K. McInnes, N. Sarajlic, J. Lavelle, I. Sarajlic, and M. P. Massagli. 1999. "Disability Associated With Psychiatric Comorbidity and Health Status in Bosnian Refugees Living in Croatia." *JAMA* 282: 433–439.

Mont, D., and Viet Cuong. 2011. "Disability and Poverty in Vietnam." *World Bank Economic Review* 25 (2): 323–359.

Nario-Redmond, M. R., J. G. Noel, and E. Fern. 2013. "Redefining Disability, Re-imagining the Self: Disability Identification Predicts Self-esteem and Strategic Responses to Stigma." *Self and Identity* 12 (5): 468–488.

Ntshangase, Sibusiso, Andile Mdikana, and Candice Cronk. 2008. "A Comparative Study of the Self-Esteem of Adolescent Boys with and without Learning Disabilities in an Inclusive School." *International Journal of Special Education* 23 (2): 75–84.

Nussbaum, Martha. 2003. "Capabilities as Fundamental Entitlements: Sen and Social Justice." *Feminist Economics* 9 (2–3): 33–59.

Pestka, K., and S. Wendt. 2014. "Belonging: Women Living with Intellectual Disabilities and Experiences of Domestic Violence." *Disability and Society* 29 (7): 1031–1045. doi:10.1080/09687599.2014.902358.

Robeyns, I. 2003. "Sen's Capability Approach and Gender Inequality: Selecting Relevant Capabilities." *Feminist Economics* 9 (2–3): 61–92. doi:10.1080/1354570022000078024.

Robeyns, I. 2006. "Three Models of Education: Rights, Capabilities and Human Capital." *Theory and Research in Education* 4 (1): 69–84.

Secrétariat d'Etat chargé de la famille, de l'enfance et des personnes handicapées. 2004. *Enquête nationale sur le handicap. Synthèse des résultats*. Rabat: Secrétariat d'Etat charge de la famille, de l'enfance et des personnes handicapées.

Sen, A. 1976. "Poverty: An Ordinal Approach to Measurement." *Econometrica* 44 (2): 219–231.

Sen, A. 1979. "Issues in the Measurement of Poverty." *Scandinavian Journal of Economics* 81 (2): 285–307.

Sen, A. 1981. *Poverty and Famines: An Essay on Entitlement and Deprivation*. Oxford: Clarendon Press, 257.

Sen, A. K. 1992. *Inequality Re-examined*. Oxford: Clarendon Press.

Sen, A. 1996. "On The Foundations of Welfare Economics: Utility, Capability and Practical Reason." In *Ethics, Rationality, and Economic Behaviour*, edited by F. Farina, F. Hahn and S. Vannucci, 50–65. Oxford: Clarendon Press.

Sen, A. K. 1999. *Development as Freedom*. Oxford: Oxford University Press.

Sen, A. 2009. *The Idea of Justice*. Cambridge, MA: The Belknap Press of Harvard University Press.

Sen, Amartya. 2002. "Why Health Equity?" *Health Economics* 11 (8): 659–666.

Trani, J. F., and P. Bakhshi. 2008. "Challenges for Assessing Disability Prevalence: The Case of Afghanistan." *ALTER European Journal of Disability Research* 2: 44–64.

Trani, J. F., and P. Bakhshi. 2011. "Profiling and Understanding People with Disabilities in Afghanistan." In *Development Effort in Afghanistan: Is There a Will and a Way? The Case of Disability and Vulnerability*, edited by J. F. Trani, 73–102. Paris: L'Harmattan.

Trani, J. F., P. Bakhshi, N. Bellanca, M. Biggeri, and F. Marchetta. 2011. "Disabilities through the Capability Approach lens: Implications for Public Policies." *European Journal of Disability Research* 5 (3): 143–157.

Trani, J. F., P. Bakhshi, and J. L. Dubois. 2006. *Understanding Vulnerability of Afghans with Disability Livelihoods, Employment, Income*. Lyon: Handicap International.

Trani, J. F., M. Biggeri, and V. Mauro. 2013. "The Multidimensionality of Child Poverty: Evidence from Afghanistan." *Social Indicators Research* 112 (2): 391–416.

Trani, J. F., J. Browne, M. Kett, O. Bah, T. Morlai, N. Bailey, and N. Groce. 2011. "Access to Health Care, Reproductive Health and Disability: A Large Scale Survey in Sierra Leone." *Social Science and Medicine* 73 (10): 1477–1489.

Trani, J. F., and T. I. Cannings. 2013. "Child Poverty in an Emergency and Conflict Context: A Multidimensional Profile and an Identification of the Poorest Children in Western Darfur." *World Development* 48: 48–70.

Trani, Jean-Francois, and Mitchell Loeb. 2012. "Poverty and Disability: A Vicious Circle? Evidence from Afghanistan and Zambia." *Journal of International Development* 24: S19–S52. doi:10.1002/jid.1709.

Tsui, K. 2002. "Multidimensional Poverty Indices." *Social Choice and Welfare* 19: 69–93.

United Nations. 2006. *Convention on the Rights of Persons with Disabilities*. New York, NY: United Nations.

Wolbring, Gregor. 1994. "Violence and Abuse in the Lives of People with Disabilities." *Aggressive Behavior* 58: 47.

World Bank. 2009. *Escaping Stigma and Neglect. People with Disabilities in Sierra Leone*. Washington, DC: World Bank.

World Health Organization, and World Bank. 2011. *World Report on Disability*. Geneva: World Health Organization.

Appendix1. Dimension weights for Morocco and Tunisia derived from two rank-to-weight methods

		Morocco		Tunisia	
Dimensions	Indicators	AD Method	DKR Method	AD Method	DKR Method
Health	Quality of health care	7.60	7.65	5.17	4.95
	Food security	6.68	6.63	9.12	9.34
Education	Access to school	6.71	6.67	6.84	6.80
	Literacy (read and write)	7.58	7.62	7.44	7.48
Employment	Access to work (18–65)	8.26	8.37	5.02	4.76
Living conditions/material wellbeing	Access to clean drinking water	6.02	5.91	9.26	9.52
	Indoor air pollution	1.71	1.43	3.02	3.04
	Type of toilet	4.01	4.29	3.23	3.28
	Type of lighting	2.09	1.90	2.82	2.81
	Overcrowding space	2.86	2.86	3.44	3.51
	Number and type of assets	3.62	3.81	1.77	1.64
Social participation	Community activities	5.94	4.76	9.21	10.71
	Friendship	8.35	9.52	5.08	3.57
Psych well-being	Depressed or anxious state	8.10	8.33	8.74	9.52
	Feeling of happiness	6.19	5.95	5.54	4.76
Physical security	Maltreatment	7.44	7.48	7.66	7.79
	Sense of security	6.84	6.80	6.63	6.49

Appendix 2. Spearman rank correlation coefficients between dimensions of deprivation

Morocco	Quality of health care	Food security	Scholl attainment/ attendance	Literacy (read and write)	Non-employment (18–65)	Access to clean drinking water	Indoor air pollution	Type of toilet	Type of lighting	Over-crowded space	Number and type of assets	Community activities	Friendship	Depressed or anxious state	Feeling of happiness	Maltreat-ment	Sense of security
Quality of health care	1																
Food security	0.14	1															
	0.00																
School attainment/ attendance	0.00	0.07	1														
	0.88	0.01															
Literacy (read and write)	0.03	0.12	0.76	1													
	0.40	0.00	0.00														
Non-employment (18–65)	0.01	0.03	0.00	0.02	1												
	0.73	0.21	0.97	0.58													
Access to clean drinking water	–0.02	0.14	0.15	0.15	–0.04	1											
	0.47	0.00	0.00	0.00	0.12												
Indoor air pollution	0.18	0.09	0.03	0.09	0.03	0.06	1										
	0.00	0.00	0.31	0.00	0.29	0.03											
Type of toilet	0.08	0.16	0.06	0.08	0.02	0.41	0.06	1									
	0.00	0.00	0.03	0.00	0.49	0.00	0.04										
Type of lighting	0.01	0.09	0.05	0.07	0.01	0.21	0.12	0.23	1								
	0.74	0.00	0.07	0.01	0.79	0.00	0.00	0.00									
Overcrowded space	0.03	0.17	–0.02	0.05	0.00	0.05	–0.02	0.11	0.00	1							
	0.29	0.00	0.41	0.09	0.91	0.06	0.59	0.00	0.90								
Number and type of assets	0.07	0.25	0.08	0.12	–0.02	0.18	0.11	0.23	0.29	0.20	1						
	0.03	0.00	0.01	0.00	0.53	0.00	0.00	0.00	0.00	0.00							
Community activities	0.05	–0.06	0.11	0.07	0.03	–0.06	0.07	–0.02	–0.01	–0.05	–0.02	1					
	0.09	0.04	0.00	0.01	0.33	0.04	0.01	0.55	0.78	0.08	0.58						
Friendship	0.07	0.15	0.23	0.26	0.09	0.03	0.11	0.07	0.00	0.05	0.09	0.25	1				

(*Continued*)

Appendix 2. Continued

Morocco	Quality of health care	Food security	Scholl attainment/ attendance	Literacy (read and write)	Non-employment (18–65)	Access to clean drinking water	Indoor air pollution	Type of toilet	Type of lighting	Over-crowded space	Number and type of assets	Community activities	Friendship	Depressed or anxious. state	Feeling of happiness	Maltreat-ment	Sense of security
	0.02	0.00	0.00	0.00	0.00	0.27	0.00	0.01	0.89	0.11	0.00	0.00					
Depressed or anxious state	0.19	0.15	0.00	0.02	0.10	–0.01	0.13	0.05	–0.01	0.02	0.03	0.18	0.23	1			
	0.00	0.00	0.96	0.39	0.00	0.80	0.00	0.06	0.76	0.52	0.38	0.00	0.00				
Feeling of happiness	0.16	0.15	0.00	0.01	0.11	0.01	0.16	0.02	–0.01	0.05	0.06	0.11	0.24	0.42	1		
	0.00	0.00	0.91	0.61	0.00	0.73	0.00	0.53	0.61	0.06	0.03	0.00	0.00	0.00			
Maltreatment	0.08	0.04	–0.09	–0.08	0.08	0.00	0.01	0.06	–0.03	0.02	0.00	0.08	0.07	0.10	0.10	1	
	0.01	0.17	0.00	0.01	0.00	0.98	0.69	0.04	0.35	0.43	0.93	0.00	0.02	0.00	0.00		
Sense of security	0.06	0.09	–0.03	0.01	0.04	–0.01	0.14	0.06	0.01	0.03	0.06	0.14	0.17	0.25	0.35	0.13	1
	0.06	0.00	0.30	0.81	0.12	0.85	0.00	0.04	0.78	0.35	0.02	0.00	0.00	0.00	0.00	0.00	

Appendix 2. Continued

Tunisia	Quality of health care	Food security	School attainment/ attendance	Literacy (read and write)	Non-employment (18–65)	Access to clean drinking water	Indoor air pollution	Type of toilet	Type of lighting	Over-crowding	Number and type of assets	Community activities	Friend-ship	Depressed or anxious state	Feeling of happiness	Maltreat-ment	Sense of security
Quality of health care	1																
Food security	0.05	1															
	0.13																
School attainment/ attendance	–0.03	0.05	1														
	0.27	0.12															
Literacy (read and write)	0.01	0.12	0.74	1													
	0.78	0.00	0.00														
Non-employment (18–65)	0.02	0.07	–0.21	–0.09	1												
	0.61	0.03	0.00	0.00													
Access to clean drinking water	0.04	0.08	0.11	0.10	0.02	1											
	0.17	0.01	0.00	0.00	0.5[illegible]												
Indoor air pollution	0.01	0.06	0.00	0.00	0.0[illegible]	0.05	1										
	0.78	0.05	0.88	0.93	0.3[illegible]	0.11											
Type of toilet	–0.02	0.13	0.15	0.12	–0.0[illegible]	0.10	0.19	1									
	0.54	0.00	0.00	0.00	0.3[illegible]	0.00	0.00										
Type of lighting	–0.04	0.05	0.08	0.08	–0.02	0.03	0.15	0.06	1								
	0.25	0.12	0.01	0.01	0.6[illegible]	0.39	0.00	0.05									
Overcrowded space	0.01	0.15	0.07	0.08	0.05	0.13	0.09	0.17	0.06	1							
	0.80	0.00	0.02	0.01	0.09	0.00	0.00	0.00	0.05								
Number and type of assets	0.07	0.24	0.14	0.18	–0.01	0.22	0.07	0.17	0.07	0.28	1						
	0.01	0.00	0.00	0.00	0.62	0.00	0.03	0.00	0.03	0.00							
Community activities	0.06	0.08	0.04	0.07	0.08	–0.05	0.02	–0.06	0.07	0.02	0.06	1					
	0.04	0.01	0.24	0.02	0.01	0.10	0.55	0.05	0.03	0.49	0.05						
Friendship	0.07	0.08	0.19	0.25	0.07	0.00	0.02	0.03	–0.01	0.04	0.03	0.24	1				
	0.02	0.01	0.00	0.00	0.02	0.96	0.61	0.25	0.67	0.19	0.27	0.00					
Depressed or anxious state	0.08	0.17	0.00	0.03	0.07	–0.03	0.02	0.01	0.00	0.07	0.06	0.13	0.14	1			
	0.01	0.00	0.95	0.27	0.02	0.27	0.41	0.83	0.92	0.03	0.03	0.00	0.00				
Feeling of happiness	0.08	0.18	0.03	0.03	0.03	–0.05	–0.01	–0.01	–0.05	0.09	0.09	0.08	0.17	0.38	1		
	0.01	0.00	0.39	0.31	0.26	0.09	0.80	0.64	0.12	0.00	0.00	0.01	0.00	0.00			
Maltreatment	0.01	0.11	–0.06	–0.08	0.07	0.01	–0.04	0.04	–0.03	0.02	0.06	–0.03	0.04	0.07	0.13	1	
	0.76	0.00	0.06	0.01	0.02	0.77	0.22	0.17	0.41	0.55	0.05	0.30	0.16	0.02	0.00		
Sense of security	0.08	0.11	–0.07	–0.09	0.03	–0.05	–0.03	0.02	–0.03	0.00	–0.05	–0.01	0.05	0.16	0.20	0.13	1
	0.01	0.00	0.03	0.00	0.31	0.11	0.38	0.43	0.27	1.00	0.11	0.65	0.08	0.00	0.00	0.00	

Appendix 3. Contribution of each dimension to poverty for various subgroups of interest

Morocco	Quality of health care	Food security	School attainment/ attendance	Literacy (read and write)	Non-employment (18–65)	Access to clean drinking water	Indoor air pollution	Type of toilet	Type of lighting	Over-crowded space	Number and type of assets	Community activities	Friend-ship	Depressed or anxious state	Feeling of happiness	Maltreat-ment	Sense of security
All	3.24	9.35	10.25	11.44	21.54	1.9	0.76	0.98	0.31	0.95	1.47	11.23	9.2	5.75	5.49	2.94	3.43
Disability status																	
Cases	3.24	9.31	9.33	10.69	19.83	1.79	0.79	0.92	0.24	0.91	1.42	11.12	9.53	7.41	6.58	3.29	3.92
Control	3.37	9.47	12.63	13.41	26.02	2.19	0.67	1.14	0.51	1.05	1.6	11.49	8.34	1.39	2.66	2.02	2.15
Gender																	
Men disabled	3.33	9.51	7.61	9.17	19.39	1.99	0.87	0.84	0.28	1.01	1.23	11.47	9.49	7.53	7.82	4.38	4.5
Men non-disabled	5.89	10.97	12.26	12.29	20.65	2.58	0.65	1.94	0.65	1.29	1.94	11.61	6.45	1.94	3.23	3.87	1.94
Women disabled	3.15	9.14	10.82	12	20.2	1.62	0.72	1	0.21	0.81	1.59	10.82	9.56	7.31	5.5	2.35	3.43
Women non-disabled	2.76	9.11	12.72	13.66	27.33	2.09	0.68	0.94	0.47	1	1.53	11.47	8.8	1.26	2.52	1.57	2.2
Age group																	
Cases below 18	4.74	9.05	7.54	12.06	0	2.51	2.01	0.5	0	2.01	2.51	10.55	10.55	7.54	12.06	9.05	7.54
Controls below 18	10.67	15.79	5.26	10.53	0	5.26	0	3.51	0	1.75	0	15.79	15.79	5.26	0	10.53	0
Cases 18–65	3.48	8.36	7.13	9.1	23.61	1.8	0.82	0.99	0.17	0.83	1	11.31	8.85	7.38	7.13	3.93	4.43
Controls 18–65	3.72	6.2	11.16	11.16	27.27	2.48	0.41	1.65	0.41	0.83	1.24	14.88	12.4	0	1.24	1.24	3.72
Cases over 65	3.12	9.57	9.97	11.03	19.69	1.76	0.73	0.92	0.27	0.88	1.48	11.1	9.66	7.41	6.21	2.88	3.64
Controls over 65	3.13	9.68	13.01	13.76	26.59	2.07	0.72	1.01	0.53	1.06	1.69	10.98	7.66	1.45	2.9	1.88	2.02
Residence																	
Rabat cases	3.72	8.95	8.46	10.64	19.59	0.73	1.21	0.24	0.16	0.77	1.65	11.73	9.67	7.28	6.89	3.26	5.32
Rabat controls	2.29	8.72	12.38	13.23	28.14	0.75	1.13	0.19	0.28	0.66	1.32	12.95	9.85	1.13	3.39	1.13	2.53

Chaouia cases	2.92	9.56	9.91	10.72	19.98	2.51	0.51	1.37	0.3	1	1.27	10.72	9.43	7.49	6.37	3.3	2.99
Chaouia controls	4.26	10.08	12.83	13.56	24.29	3.36	0.31	1.91	0.69	1.38	1.83	10.31	7.1	1.6	2.06	2.75	1.83
Type of disability																	
Non-disabled	3.37	9.47	12.63	13.41	26.02	2.19	0.67	1.14	0.51	1.05	1.6	11.49	8.34	1.39	2.66	2.02	2.15
Moderate disability	3.66	10.66	8.72	10.18	21.32	1.29	0.81	1.29	0.16	0.48	1.97	11.15	7.27	7.75	3.88	5.33	4.36
Physical	1.98	11.28	10.57	12.22	20.67	2.13	0.55	1.02	0.55	1.19	1.83	10.34	8.93	6.58	5.64	2.35	2.35
Sensory	3.5	8.63	5.28	8.54	21.14	1.63	1.08	1.08	0.41	0.68	1.63	10.98	10.57	7.72	7.32	4.07	6.1
Intellectual and mental	4.42	11.09	8.07	10.59	20.17	1.71	0.67	1.18	0	0.84	1.85	9.58	9.08	8.57	6.55	2.02	4.03
Multiple	3.43	8	10.18	10.69	18.76	1.82	0.84	0.71	0.13	0.94	0.99	11.8	10.08	7.39	7.36	3.33	3.95
Tunisia																	
All	2.42	7.07	8.87	11.91	24.18	0.6	0.09	0.45	0.09	0.87	1.91	13.07	9.13	6	6.18	4.57	2.6
Disability status																	
Cases	1.87	6.79	8.43	11.25	22.49	0.47	0.12	0.39	0.08	0.94	1.84	13.12	9.61	7.15	7.61	5.04	2.81
Controls	4.18	7.98	10.27	14.07	29.66	1.01	0	0.63	0.13	0.63	2.15	12.93	7.6	2.28	1.52	3.04	1.9
Gender																	
Men disabled	2.34	6.73	5.85	10.24	25.76	0.68	0	0.29	0	1.37	1.95	13.17	8.49	7.02	8.49	5.56	2.05
Men non-disabled	12.37	6.19	6.19	9.28	24.74	0	0	0	0	0	1.03	12.37	9.28	6.19	6.19	3.09	3.09
Women disabled	1.56	6.84	10.16	11.91	20.31	0.33	0.2	0.46	0.13	0.65	1.76	13.09	10.35	7.23	7.03	4.69	3.32
Women non-disabled	3.03	8.24	10.84	14.74	30.35	1.16	0	0.72	0.14	0.72	2.31	13.01	7.37	1.73	0.87	3.03	1.73
Age group																	
Cases below 18	7.89	0	15.79	15.79	0	0	0	0	0	2.63	2.63	15.79	7.89	7.89	15.79	7.89	0
Controls below 18	NA	NA	NA	NA	NA	NA	NA	NA	Na	NA	NA	NA	NA	NA	NA	NA	NA
Cases 18–65	1.76	6.6	6.74	10.26	28.14	0.49	0.05	0.2	0.05	0.93	1.71	13.04	8.94	6.3	6.6	5.57	2.64

(Continued)

Appendix 3. Continued

Morocco	Quality of health care	Food security	School attainment/ attendance	Literacy (read and write)	Non-employment (18–65)	Access to clean drinking water	Indoor air pollution	Type of toilet	Type of lighting	Over-crowded space	Number and type of assets	Community activities	Friend-ship	Depressed or anxious state	Feeling of happiness	Maltreat-ment	Sense of security
Controls 18–65	3.89	8.17	10.12	14.01	30.35	1.04	0	0.65	0.13	0.65	2.2	12.84	7.39	2.33	1.56	2.72	1.95
Cases over 65	1.89	8.19	15.13	15.13	0	0.42	0.42	1.26	0.21	0.84	2.31	13.24	12.61	10.71	11.34	2.52	3.78
Controls over 65	16.67	0	16.67	16.67	0	0	0	0	0	0	0	16.67	16.67	0	0	16.67	0
Residence																	
Tunis cases	1.63	7.75	7.95	10.81	22.43	0	0	0.07	0.07	0.48	1.29	13.66	8.97	8.36	8.57	4.69	3.26
Tunis controls	3.2	11.74	6.41	12.81	29.89	0.36	0	0	0.36	0	1.07	13.88	9.61	3.2	2.14	3.2	2.14
Béja cases	2.2	5.5	9.08	11.83	22.57	1.1	0.28	0.83	0.09	1.56	2.57	12.39	10.46	5.5	6.33	5.5	2.2
Béja controls	4.72	5.91	12.4	14.76	29.53	1.38	0	0.98	0	0.98	2.76	12.4	6.5	1.77	1.18	2.95	1.77
Type of disability																	
Non-disabled	4.18	7.98	10.27	14.07	29.66	1.01	0	0.63	0.13	0.63	2.15	12.93	7.6	2.28	1.52	3.04	1.9
Moderate disability	2.01	9.03	6.02	7.02	26.09	0	0.33	0.67	0.33	1	2.34	12.04	9.03	6.02	7.02	8.03	3.01
Physical	1.65	8.81	7.16	12.11	22.02	0.37	0.18	0.73	0	1.65	2.94	13.76	5.5	9.91	7.16	4.4	1.65
Sensory	2.94	5.88	14.71	14.71	23.53	1.96	0	0	0	0.98	0	11.76	11.76	2.94	5.88	2.94	0
Intellectual and mental	1.69	7.58	4.21	10.11	25.28	0.84	0.28	0.28	0	0	2.53	13.48	8.43	5.06	8.43	6.74	5.06
Multiple	1.91	5.24	10.25	11.91	20.97	0.4	0	0.24	0.08	0.87	1.19	13.11	11.68	7.15	7.86	4.29	2.86

Corporate Contributions to Developing Health Capabilities

REGINA MOCZADLO, HARALD STROTMANN & JÜRGEN VOLKERT

ABSTRACT *Despite the importance of the private sector for global development, few researchers have analyzed corporate impacts on capabilities and sustainable human development (SHD).*[1] *Our article aims to contribute to an improved understanding of corporate potentials, impacts and risks for SHD. More specifically, we concentrate on health and health capabilities and exemplify our arguments based on our evaluation of health initiatives in the Bayer CropScience's Model Village Project (MVP). Based on representative primary quantitative survey data for two model and two control villages, as well as qualitative studies, we explain and analyze the corporate health-related activities in the model villages. We discuss how these corporate initiatives might fit into a business case, examine how they have changed the well-being of the populace as reported by the villagers, and provide results on stakeholder trust. Furthermore, we reconsider the risks of corporate neglect or even violation of important health issues. We conclude with lessons learned from the MVP and with consequences for subsequent capability approach research.*

1. Introduction

When doing business in developing countries, it is generally expected that multinational companies (MNC) will generate employment and income as well as create technology and productivity spillovers (Blalock and Gertler 2008; Iršová and Havránek 2013; Smeets 2008). However, it has been shown by development studies that a variety of further well-being dimensions and means are important for people's well-being, which may be improved, neglected or violated by MNCs (Scherer and Palazzo 2011).

Schölmerich (2013, 29–30) used the CA to analyze the consequences of companies' corporate social responsibility (CSR) initiatives on poverty reduction in Cambodia. She found that the evaluated CSR measures from the private sector have positive effects on their stakeholders. Furthermore, she found built-in CSR strategies—where companies include CSR activities in their core business—to be more effective than bolt-on strategies without a connection to the core business. With the "Model Village Project" (MVP), Bayer CropScience follows a built-in strategy. While doing business with smallholder farmers, who are suppliers selling cotton seeds, the firm began to implement measures that can both contribute to sustainable human development (SHD) in the villages and improve the long-term performance of the company's supply chain. The authors of this article provide an independent evaluation for the MVP. The evaluation strategy presented here is based upon the capability approach (CA) (Volkert, Strotmann, and Moczadlo 2014).

The focus of the people-centered CA lies in the capabilities and real freedoms that people value and have reason to value (Sen [1999] 2000). Therefore, the evaluation of Bayer CropScience's impacts on the development of health capabilities (Ruger 1998, 2004) begins with an analysis of the values that the villagers attach to their health capability and with an examination of their perceptions of health-related freedoms, restrictions and potentials for improvement. Subjective health perceptions are important to identify individual suffering. However, they can be severely misleading as a result of adaptation to social experiences and circumstances. Therefore, we mirror these subjective findings with the objective health and nutrition data.

As the MVP initiatives began only a few years ago, this article describes a work in progress. It is organized as follows: Section 2 briefly describes the role of health in the CA, based predominantly on Sen and Ruger. The first applications of the capability approach to health and health care were developed by Ruger (1998, 2003, 2004, 2006a, 2006b, 2007a, 2007b, 2008a, 2008b) and Ruger and Kim (2006), starting nearly two decades ago. This pioneering work created the field of capabilities and health, generating its own secondary literature. Since that time, Ruger's lines of reasoning and program of work has expanded significantly to provide theoretical and empirical resources for this and other studies. In Section 3, the aims and motivations of the MVP and Bayer CropScience in terms of health-related investments are characterized. Section 4 explains the methodology for the evaluation of the MVP and the data used, while Section 5 analyzes the subjective and objective health situation of the villagers and the gaps between the situations. Section 6 describes the corporate activities that have already begun in the model villages to enhance health capabilities and, thereby, also discusses opportunities and threats in the implementation process. Based on empirical evidence, Section 7 discusses the possible positive contributions by the corporate activities on the development of health capabilities, but also their problems, limitations and risks. Section 8 concludes with lessons learned and with consequences for subsequent CA research.

2. Health in the CA

2.1. Concepts of Health and Health Capabilities

Health is valuable in and of itself (Ruger 1998, 2003, 2004). Further, it is an instrument for vitality (Alkire and Santos 2014, 253). Health also has a major instrumental influence on one's capability to participate in economic and social life (Sen 1992, 44). Good nutrition is a prerequisite for the capability to live a long and healthy life and is a central element of human freedom. The World Health Organization (WHO) defines health as "... a state of complete physical, mental and social well-being and not merely the absence of disease or infirmity" (UN 1947, 29).

Health is not only constitutive of the well-being of people but also an enabler for people to function as agents, in the sense of realizing the goals they have reason to value (Anand 2004; Ruger 1998, 2004, 18). People's options to realize freedoms and capabilities depend on their health achievements (Ruger 1998, 2004; Sen 2002, 660).

Sen (2002, 660) distinguishes "… between health achievement and the *capability* to achieve good health … " and evaluates, in this context, health achievement as "… a good guide … " for the existing capabilities. He is convinced that people will decide in favor of good health if they have real opportunity of choice. Sen (2008) and Ruger (2006b) perceive health as a human right that has several influencing factors, such as "… nutrition, lifestyle, education, women's empowerment, and the extent of inequality and unfreedom in a society."

Ruger (2010, 47) defines health capability as the: "Confidence and ability to be effective in achieving optimal health [by] given biologic and genetic disposition; intermediate and broader social, political, and economic environment; and access to the public health and health care system." Hence, the concept of health capability is broader than health and health functioning—it is the outcome of health choices. For Ruger, besides health outcomes, health capability includes also health agency (2009, 3).

2.2. Determinants of Health Capabilities

An important characteristic of the CA is the emphasis on the freedom of choice out of a capability set that people have for their own well-being (Leßmann 2013, 26; Sen [1999] 2000, 73). People have good reasons to value a self-determined life and to have personal agency over their own life and surroundings (Halpern et al. 2004, 7). In the CA literature, a consensus has emerged that personal freedom implies personal responsibility (Fleurbaey 2002, 74). Lifestyle and behavior influence the health outcomes of people as much as the health care system does (Halpern et al. 2004, 6).

The concept of health capability (Ruger 2010) allows for the analysis of the conditions that, on the one hand, stimulate and, on the other hand, hamper the ability of people to make health choices. It includes both internal factors like health knowledge (i.e. health-seeking skills and beliefs) and health values as well as external factors like social norms, material circumstances or economic, political and social security. Health capability further has consequences for diverse individuals' freedoms, among them self-management or knowledge and competences (Ruger 2010, 41–46).

Adaptation to social circumstances but also a lack of education, missing available health facilities and a lack of public information on illness and remedies often cause misperceptions of one's own health status in poor, rural parts of the developing world (Vellakkal et al. 2013, 5–10). As Sen (2009, 285–286) puts it:

> The internal view of the patient may be seriously limited by his or her knowledge and social experience. A person reared in a community with great many diseases and little medical facilities may be inclined to take certain symptoms as 'normal' when they are clinically preventable.

As such, it is theoretically well-established and an empirically frequent phenomenon to find gaps between the objective health status of people and their subjective health perception (Sen 2009, 284–290).

Alkire (2010) emphasizes the importance of differentiating between instrumental freedoms, the social and environmental conversion factors, and intrinsic freedoms, which are valuable in themselves. Social actors like MNCs provide instrumental freedoms. In an evaluation of a company's sustainability strategy, the consequences of improved instrumental freedoms on the real freedoms of people have to be taken into account (Volkert, Strotmann, and Moczadlo 2014, 4).

According to Ruger (2010, 42–43, 1998), society has an obligation to provide adequate conditions for everyone so that they are enabled to be healthy. This implies that health capability gaps are reduced through interventions both on individual and societal levels. This is important because the health choices that people can make depend on the capability sets people can choose from, which are influenced by the factors mentioned above. To ignore these influencing factors would mean to hold people responsible for outcomes over which they do not have, or only partly have, control (Ruger 2010; Venkatapuram 2011, 22). Ruger (2008b, 423–433) further calls for a "shared health governance" between states and institutions and mentions business as an actor for "… sharing responsibility to correct global health injustice". Nonetheless, governments shoulder the main responsibility for health justice, because private institutions "… lack sufficient incentive and ability to undertake population-wide measures … " (Ng and Ruger 2014, 287). The Health Capability Paradigm (HCP) (Ruger 2009) examines health—and non-health—sector variables.

Ruger's (2010, 42) focus is on health capabilities because she sees them as a means to address the essential balance between paternalism and autonomy. However, governance gaps and government failures more and more have the consequence that MNCs as well as other stakeholder groups are taking over societal tasks (Moczadlo and Volkert 2012).[2]

The development of human resources is an important challenge for the global private sector due to the restricted resources of states. In this context, the development and enhancement of capabilities become de facto more and more a topic for private companies. Cameron and Eyeson (2012, 176), reffering to Sen, state that from a CA perspective, people may profit from companies' measures not only by receiving a higher income and productivity increase but also by other elements of substantive freedoms.

The MPV is an example of an activity by a MNC that plans to implement health measures as part of its social supply chain management and thus aims to contribute to closing the health-related governance gaps. The intention of the company is to create a win-win-situation for both the smallholder farmers and Bayer CropScience. Lack of sanitation and hygiene causes some 4% of the global burden of (mostly) diarrheal diseases. Malnutrition and malaria, which are also prevalent in rural areas, account for more than 3% of the global burden of diseases (WWAP 2012, 725). For Bayer CropScience, this reduces the productivity of corporate suppliers and their families (see, e.g. Asenso-Okyere et al. 2011, 10). For families, low productivity leads to low income and the lack of investment potential for productivity increasing investment. For Bayer, restricted productivity results in a persistent lack of supply chain competitiveness.

From a business case perspective, the health and nutrition investments of MNCs are thus means for improving farmers' potential to work and invest in human capital. Health investments can thus directly improve a person's productivity; furthermore, they complement investments in education and physical capital (Ruger et al. 2012, 760).

A comprehensive literature review of Walters and James (2009, 7), however, shows that it is relatively uncommon to find proactive and voluntary improvements of the health of suppliers and employees by large producers in the global supply chain. The cases they identified for positive influences through buyers were mostly motivated by external pressures from companies' stakeholders, which created reputational risks.

2.3. Trust as Prerequisite for Changing Health Preferences and Successful Business

The term "trust" can be defined "… as the psychological willingness of a party to be vulnerable to the actions of another party (individual or organization) based on positive expectations regarding the other party's motivation and/or behavior" (Pirson and Malhotra 2011, 1088). Organizational trust is an enabler for business efficiency and success. It may foster cooperation within companies and between corporate stakeholders. Trust can promote commitment, serve as a motivator and result in more creativity, innovation, knowledge transfer and competitive advantages.

However, trust in business has been violated by the diverse scandals of and unethical behaviors by business executives, due to personal greed and/or the enormous pressure to increase a company's value (Clapham et al. 2014, 55). As such, businesses currently have to gain credibility as a prerequisite for business cases.

Trust building and effective communication are also prerequisites for the establishment of successful long-term relations in the supply chain, and personal relations improve business ties when dealing with farmers (Fischer 2013, p. 213). In the literature, trust and the trust-building processes are often described with the dimensions ability, benevolence and integrity (e.g. Mayer, Davis, and Schoorman 1995). Ability consists of the skills and competences the business partner has. Integrity means that a contract partner will fulfill his/her obligations as promised. Benevolence is the expectation that a business partner will do something good for the supplier aside from pure profit motives (Schoorman et al. 2007, 345). Pirson and Malhotra (2011) find that trust in companies is relationship-specific and differs widely across different types of stakeholders. External stakeholders, like suppliers, with shallow relationships base trust on the perception of integrity, whereas in a deep relationship, trust is based on benevolence (Pirson and Malhotra 2011, 1099), notably on the corporation's concern, care and interest with respect to their stakeholders' well-being (Pirson and Malhotra 2011, 1092). Pirson and Milhotra (2011, 1100) also mention the limitations of their study. They emphasize that beyond the Western European stakeholders that they addressed, major differences in other institutional and cultural contexts, as well as an asymmetry of dependence, may have an impact on suppliers' trust. These issues are important in a rural Indian context. Contrary to well-educated Western European stakeholders, almost half of the population is illiterate (Volkert, Strotmann, and Moczadlo 2014, 35) and extremely poor (45% of the villagers are not able to personally spend more than $1.25 per day-Volkert, Strotmann, and Moczadlo 2014, 17). They lack information as well as the human and financial capital to perform successfully from a western corporate perspective. Moreover, the relationship between the corporation and the smallholder farmers in its supply chain is characterized by a strong asymmetry in dependence. For transnational corporations, one new supplier out of thousands may fall into the category of a shallow relationship. However, if the company does not buy the harvest from a poor farmer due to a lack of contracted quality or other reasons, this may ruin the farmer. As such, when contracting with an unknown multinational company, poor farmers suffer from high uncertainty. Many poor Indian farmers are already too vulnerable to place their trust in accepting even more vulnerability by contracting with powerful transnational corporations. Therefore, MNCs may first have to create positive expectations. These can include initiatives that foster what people find valuable as well as improved preconditions for fulfilling potential contracts with large companies. Corporate health initiatives may qualify as this kind of initiative and may be seen as "strategic corporate benevolence", which can provide positive experiences for their new business partners and at the same time increase their productivity. This is most important in the beginning of a relationship when a supplier has little information about the trustee's benevolence and is dependent on the positive or negative experiences business partners make with one another (Vanneste, Puranam, and Kretschmer 2014, 1898).

Moreover, trust is also essential for the cooperation and responsiveness of poor villagers to corporate awareness rising in the domain of health and nutrition.

3. Bayer Cropscience's MVP

3.1. Background[3]

Since 2000, the Bayer AG has voluntarily committed itself to an explicit zero child labor policy and has become one of the first signatories of the United Nations Global Compact (Bayer 2014). In 2002, the company had acquired the French Corporation Aventis. Proagro, a subsidiary of Aventis, was dealing in cotton seed production in rural India. A few weeks later, in 2003, non-governmental organizations (NGOs) put pressure on Bayer CropScience to stop child labor in the fields of the supplying Indian farmers. These challenges led to an intensive and long learning process on how to apply measures to avoid child labor; a process that was eventually successful several years later: The NGOs that had accused Bayer CropScience acknowledged the company's contributions toward diminishing child labor (Subramanian 2011, 7). Due to this success, the company planned to go further and began to outline a community development strategy: the MVP.

3.2. Aims and Motivation

In an internal communication of Bayer CropScience, the goal of the Model Village Project (MVP) was specified as follows: The project is aiming at "... development of the villages in a clear win-win context by developing economically sustainable business in a triple bottom line perspective, by also providing and preserving social and environmental bottom lines". Hence, the main aim of the MVP is to explore measures that show economic and social effectiveness and efficiency. At the same time, they have to enhance people's capabilities and agency.

Two model and two control villages in rural Karnataka (South India) were selected in areas where the company was not sourcing at the time. Bayer CropScience has since initiated activities in the two model villages that can have impacts on the Bayer suppliers' value added and SHD in these villages.

4. Evaluation Methodology and Database

The scientific evaluation of the MVP applies a combination of quantitative and qualitative methods. As the evaluation concept is based on the CA, both the quantitative and the qualitative evaluations cover a wide range of information on very different aspects of well-being. In the following part of this section, details will focus on health-related aspects.

For the quantitative evaluation, a representative panel survey was implemented, both on the household and on the individual level, in the two model and two control villages of rural Karnataka. For the baseline survey in 2011, more than 2300 individuals were interviewed across almost 1000 households. Therefore, 75% of all households in the villages and households from all social background (upper castes, other castes, scheduled castes and scheduled tribes) are covered in the data in a representative manner. From August 2014 to October 2014, the 2nd wave of the panel survey was conducted. In the 2nd wave, more than 1040 households and more than 2400 individuals were interviewed, of which approximately 940 panel households (i.e. 97% of those) had already been surveyed in 2011.

As Sen (2008, 273) and Ruger (2004) emphasize the need to assess functionings and capabilities to function to take account of peoples' well-being, the questionnaire of the quantitative baseline study asked, inter alia, for the value that respondents attach to health, nutrition and other dimensions of well-being. Those interviewees who say they attach an extremely high value to health issues (i.e. to having enough food to eat) are also asked whether they feel restricted in achieving these goals.

To identify why people attach a high or a low value to diverse dimensions of well-being and the consequences they experience when lacking certain capabilities or functionings (e.g. health), structured focus group discussions (FGD) were conducted in the MVP as a qualitative assessment method, which is often proposed for the operationalization of the CA (e.g. Biggeri and Ferrannini 2014, 61; Feldman et al. 2015). Furthermore, FGD are critical to give a voice to the villagers with respect to potential ways forward. Therefore, some 250 villagers participated in 18 FGDs between 2012 and 2014. In general, 10–15 participants joined a FGD with a time frame of around 1.5 hours. Depending on the purpose, most focus groups were segmented according to gender and social background. Group sessions were tape recorded and transcribed. Categorization of information and identification of patterns were done during the field stage, based on the tape recordings and the transcripts as well as on private records, FGD drawings, dynamics of the discussion, etc.

FGDs help in understanding the quantitative results and in exposing/exploring hidden issues. For instance, a lack of information and adaptation in the domain of health was indicated in the quantitative survey and then more precisely identified and discussed in the FGDs. Another example is the lack of trust in general, and in MNCs in particular, which was brought up and further specified in the FGDs, and so trust issues could be included and analyzed into specific questions in the second quantitative panel wave.

In general, these subjective views of the respondents on health-related issues are important for identifying human suffering, which may occur irrespective of concrete objective health problems. Moreover, contrasting subjective opinions and objective findings can help to explore misperceptions and misplaced optimism. Therefore, analyses of the health status and health risks in a village should also focus on objective indicators (Ruger 1998, 2004; Ruger and Kim 2006). Within the MVP, health camps were conducted in which medical doctors from different disciplines and a team of laboratory technicians examined the health status of the inhabitants in one of the model villages. With a body mass index (BMI)[4] measurement, the nutritional status of a person can be assessed, and so the weight and height of each of the villagers were measured after every interview of the quantitative surveys. In correspondence with UNDP practices, access to safe drinking water has been operationalized as the "proportion of population using an improved drinking water source" (UN Millennium Project 2005, xix) and "the proportion of population using an improved sanitation facility" has been used for measuring access to sanitation (e.g. UNDP 2010).

5. Empirics: Objective and Subjective Assessment of the Health Situation

5.1. Subjective Health Evaluation of the Villagers

9 out of 10 villagers interviewed in our baseline study reported that the freedom to live a long and healthy life and to have enough good food is important or extremely important for a good life. Almost every fourth respondent says that he or she perceives having enough food to eat and to live a long and healthy life as extremely important.

As Figure 1 shows, almost all the people for whom the capabilities to live a long and healthy life or to be well-nourished are extremely important believe that they have the

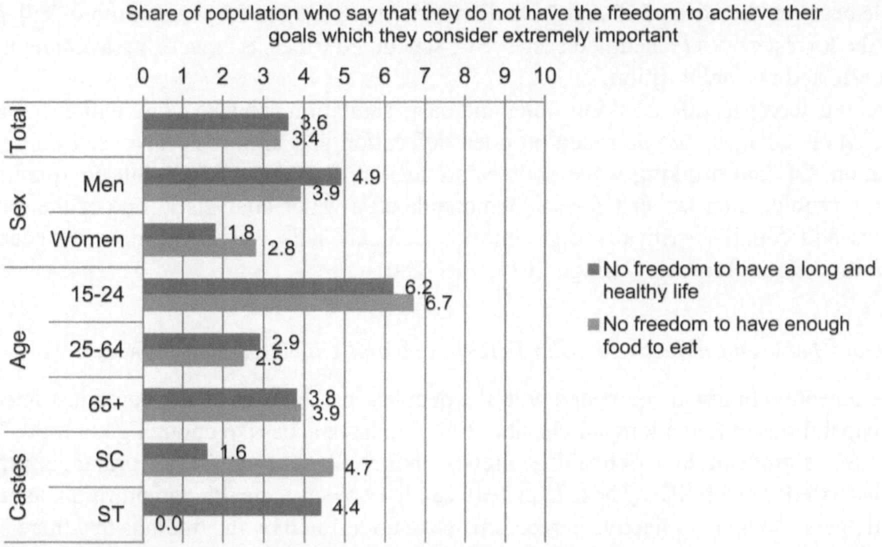

Figure 1. Subjective health evaluation of the villagers (number in percentages). *Castes*: SC: scheduled castes, ST: scheduled tribes.
Source: Model Village Project Baseline Survey, 2011, $N = 537$.

freedom to achieve this. The shares of villagers who feel deprived in these two respects are only 3% or 4% in total. Furthermore, for men and women, and for different age groups and different castes, the corresponding shares are extremely low. For villagers who belong to the lowest caste of scheduled tribes, there was not even a single villager for whom having enough food is extremely important who answered that he/she feels deprived in this respect.

This impression from the quantitative survey, that the villagers do not feel deprived with respect to health, was confirmed within the FGD, where villagers reported having no serious problems with staying in good health and getting enough good food. For instance, a male focus group of upper and lower castes unanimously agreed that they were all in good health. Only less than 10% of people in the MVP said that they do not have access to an improved water source.

5.2. Objective Assessment

Doctors in the health camps observed anemia to be common among children and adults. Quite a few of the villagers were found to be using medicines haphazardly without proper medical consultation, which can lead to a number of diseases. More than 7 in 10 people had the habit of consuming tobacco, which causes oral and dental diseases. Approximately 80% suffered from chronic generalized periodontics, 60% from dental calculus and 40% from stains. Furthermore, doctors emphasized that negligence about health is the cause behind various health problems. Hygiene was also very poor because of a lack of awareness.

Many of the diverse health issues in the villages seem to be caused by widespread malnutrition. Malnutrition causes lower resistance to infections and hence a higher prevalence of diseases (Agulanna et al. 2013, 2). According to our baseline study and the BMI measurements, nearly 45% of the population aged 15 years or older were malnourished in 2011. Women were more often affected than men, and the relationship between age and malnutrition seems to be U-shaped: malnutrition was above average for young people between the ages of 15 and 24 and for older people aged 65 years or more. Villagers from the lowest castes (scheduled castes, SC; scheduled tribes, ST) were, on average, more often affected by malnutrition.

Lacking access to safe drinking water and basic sanitation can also cause major diseases. In the MVP villages, people relied on open defecation and almost no one used improved sanitation. Official drinking water sources are available in the villages, but the quality of water is problematic: Bayer CropScience mandated a water analysis in one of the model villages and found a critically high fluoride content. This can create diseases such as dental or skeletal fluorosis (Nriagu 2011, 776–780)

5.3. Gaps between Subjective Health Perceptions and Objective Health Status

These objective findings contrasted with the peoples' perceptions of not being restricted in their capabilities to live a long and healthy life or to have access to enough good food. This indicated a significant lack of health awareness in the villages, which was further confirmed and discussed in the FGDs. These gaps between the objective health and nutrition status of the villagers and their subjective perceptions were underlined by the findings that there is no significant difference in the subjective health assessments between people who are malnourished and those who are not.

In summary, subjective health perceptions may indicate issues of suffering but are not sufficient for a reliable analysis. In particular, those who have minimal access to information and health care may wrongly suppose themselves to be in good health. As such, the low deprivation values in Figure 1, for example for ST, may only reflect adaptation and lack of information rather than good health and nutrition.

Sen (1981, p. 438) noted that people may subjectively feel that they need less food than is objectively required, which results in satisfied, though malnourished, villagers. Lack of information (ignorance), fixed food habits, or apathy may be reasons for these misperceptions. In the FGDs, the villagers stated that hunger is no longer a problem in the villages, although it had been a problem about a decade previously. Hence, the conclusion could be that, currently, as more—though still not sufficient—food is available, villagers may wrongly assume that the quantity of food is sufficient. Quite a few FGDs with women and men showed that most villagers were aware of the composition of healthy food. Nonetheless, the diet of the village people contains predominantly staple food. This may be partly because the people stated that they eat what they are used to. Some bought vegetables once a week in the market but could not store them for a week. Only a few stated that they were not able to afford healthy food.

5.4. Health Misperceptions: Consequences for SHD and Corporate Strategy

The kind of instrumental and agency-related importance that health has for the villagers has to be evaluated, in the first place, by the villagers themselves. To understand how the above mentioned misperceptions and lack of information can affect people's capabilities, lives and SHD, villagers for whom health is one of the most important dimensions of their well-being were asked for the reasons.

On the one hand, the villagers highlighted a number of instrumental issues, such as the importance of health for their ability to work, to perform productively, and to avoid financial stress like treatment costs. On the other hand, people also emphasized agency- and responsibility-related aspects of health. Notably, women explained how critical it is for them and their children to stay healthy. This is said to be of particular concern when husbands fail to fulfill their responsibilities, such as in the case of diseases or widespread alcoholism. Furthermore, a close relationship was mentioned between physical and mental health. In general, the villagers said that they perceive health as a major precondition "to achieve something in our life".

As discussed above, a company might have strategic incentives to explore ways to overcome the gap of subjective perceptions and objective conditions to reduce health risks and improve health awareness and conditions. However, gaining effective cooperation is a challenge in the villages. The 2014 MVP survey reveals that a majority of the villagers in the model and control villages (51%) distrust MNCs in general. Only less than one third (31%) of the village populations at least "rather agree" to trust MNC, while 17% are not decided on this issue.

Building trust is thus a major prerequisite for effective awareness raising and health activities by MNCs. Moreover, as the people attached a high value to health and good food, Bayer CropScience may also have gained trust with its early contributions to health and other dimensions of well-being in 2011. As such, health activities may be suitable in an early stage of corporate projects to enhance the villagers' well-being, particularly when trust still has to be established. In the following, we discuss the health-related initiatives that Bayer CropScience has implemented in the MVP.

6. Implementation of Health-Related Measures

6.1. Development Coordinator and Women's Self-Help Groups as Core Elements

Soon after the start of the MVP, it became clear that the multi-dimensionality of SHD and the resulting complexity and interdependency of SHD contributions made it impossible for Bayer CropScience to coordinate a successful strategy from a remote, urban corporate desktop. Therefore, in 2013, Bayer CropScience installed a development coordinator from a regional NGO in the model villages to advise and support the villagers. The central task of this manager was the initiation and guidance of self-help groups for women (SHGs), which have been established across all castes and which have proved elsewhere to potentially foster the empowerment of rural women in India (e.g. Deininger and Liu 2013; Feldman et al. 2015). Bayer CropScience also considers SHGs to be a device to gain trust and learn about the experiences of the villagers via the development coordinator. Within the SHGs, women collect their savings and use them for micro loans to group members, which increase the person's income and ability to accumulate capital for investment. As will be explained below, the SHGs also serve as a platform for awareness-raising workshops and measures.

6.2. Health Camps

As mentioned earlier, several health camps were organized by Bayer CropScience in one of the model villages from 2012 onwards. The first of them, in which 856 people participated, mainly served a diagnostic purpose to clarify in more detail the gap between the subjective perceptions and the objective health situation and risks. Further health camps had a stronger focus on treatment.

6.3. Water Purification

In 2011, Bayer CropScience had already initiated the installation of a water purification plant in one model village. The plant reduces the water's fluoride content and also works as an anti-bacterial device.

The water is sold (for 1 INR/10 liters) to economize its use and to avoid the need for permanent subsidies, which might make it impossible to sustainably pass over the project ownership from Bayer to the population at a later stage. Users of the purified water reported suffering less from a variety of symptoms, such as joint pain, to which they had become accustomed when relying on the consumption of the official water. However, in the first few years, only a limited share of the households bought the clean water more or less regularly. FGDs showed that technical problems - which could be overcome in the meantime - practical concerns, and mainly a lack of awareness turned out to be major obstacles for a more widespread acceptance of clean water drinking. In the FGDs, several villagers stated that they considered both kinds of water to be exact substitutes and thus were not prepared to pay for the water. After December 2013, awareness-raising activities were begun in the women's SHG. The development coordinator informed the SHG members about the potential benefits of the purified water.

6.4. Malaria Control Initiative

Karnataka's governmental health department aims to fight malaria. However, the administration that is responsible for this measure faces the problem of approaching the villagers and getting their permission to spray inside the houses. In both model villages, Bayer organized awareness workshops about malaria risks, which were conducted by health education officers from the government. In May 2014, the health department undertook the spraying of the inside and outside of the houses.

6.5. Dental Health Camp

In 2014, Bayer CropScience organized the first dental camp for schoolchildren, run by a dental college. Twelve dentists visited both model villages. School headmasters invited parents to a workshop in which dentists explained the consequences of lacking dental hygiene and the resulting illnesses. All of the parents agreed to send their children to a check-up in which their stains were removed and other minor dental illnesses were cured. Children suffering from major dental problems were or will be treated in nearby hospitals (costs covered by Bayer CropScience). All of the children received a toothbrush and toothpaste. Check-up dental health camps are planned every six months.

7. Corporate Health Initiatives' Impacts on Individual Well-being and Agency

7.1. Potentials: from Strengthened Instrumental Freedoms to Well-being and Trust

With health-related activities, Bayer CropScience has strengthened the villagers' social opportunities; most notably, their access to health care and to mitigation of health risks. Transparency guarantees have been improved by awareness raising as well as by corporate support of government programs. Nevertheless, Alkire (2010) has emphasized that such contributions to instrumental freedoms do not necessarily end in improved well-being and agency. The villagers determine whether Bayer CropScience's contributions to instrumental freedoms (particularly in the domain of health) are valued and have a real impact on the beings and doings that the people value (Volkert, Strotmann, and Moczadlo 2014). However, there is a criticism that corporate strategies at the base of the pyramid are rarely evaluated or, if so, are evaluated mainly with respect to corporate issues (costs, value added, etc.) or based on experts' opinions. The voices of the poor who are

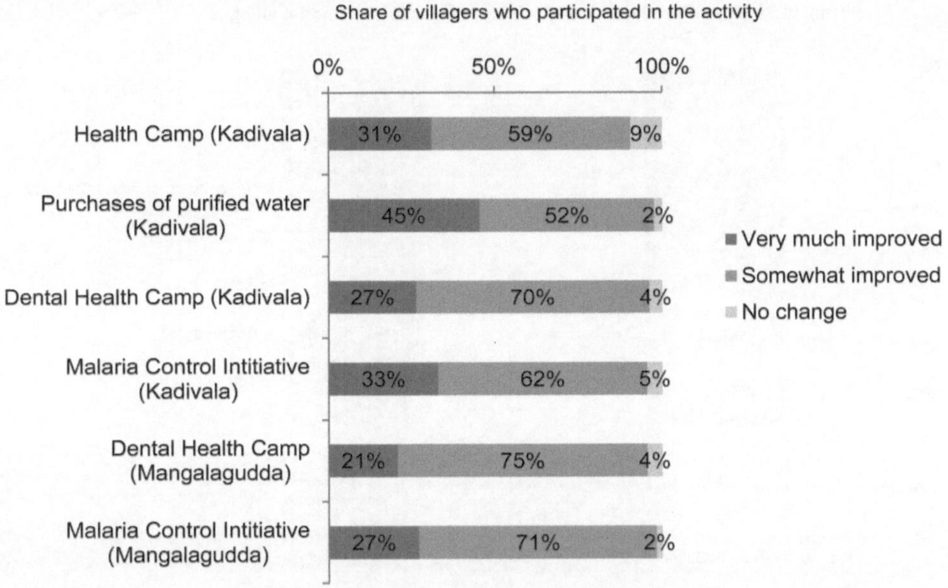

Figure 2. Perceived impacts of Bayer CropScience's initiatives on personal well-being.
Source: Model Village Project Survey, 2014, $N = 865$.

supposed to benefit from these strategies and who should be in the center of human development are mostly neglected (Schölmerich 2013). To address this drawback, villagers were explicitly asked in the quantitative MVP survey in 2014 whether and how the health-related activities of Bayer CropScience have impacted their well-being. Figure 2 shows the results.

The results illustrate that the majority of the participants saw an improvement of their overall well-being due to the health-related measures. It remains to be clarified whether these subjective perceptions of well-being can be confirmed by objective findings. Moreover, it is important to learn more about the potential critique from non-participants and non-users to gain a full picture of the potential impacts on people's well-being.

With respect to the aim of trust building, perceived positive impacts on overall individual well-being do not necessarily turn into trust. Therefore, in the quantitative MVP survey in 2014, people were also asked whether they would agree that they place trust in MNCs in general and in Bayer CropScience specifically.

As Figure 3 indicates, Bayer CropScience's health-related and other measures not only have the potential to improve self-perceived individual well-being (Figure 2) but also to raise trust in the company to a level that is substantially above the low level of trust in MNCs in general. Further quantitative analyses and FGDs will have to show which of Bayer's measures have contributed the most toward overcoming the challenge of trust building, as well as why and how this was the case.

7.2. Problems, Risks and Limitations

Up to now, our findings have shown that an MNC like Bayer CropScience can indeed help in overcoming state and market failures by providing awareness, information and access to health care, thereby reducing information asymmetries and helping people to improve their well-being.

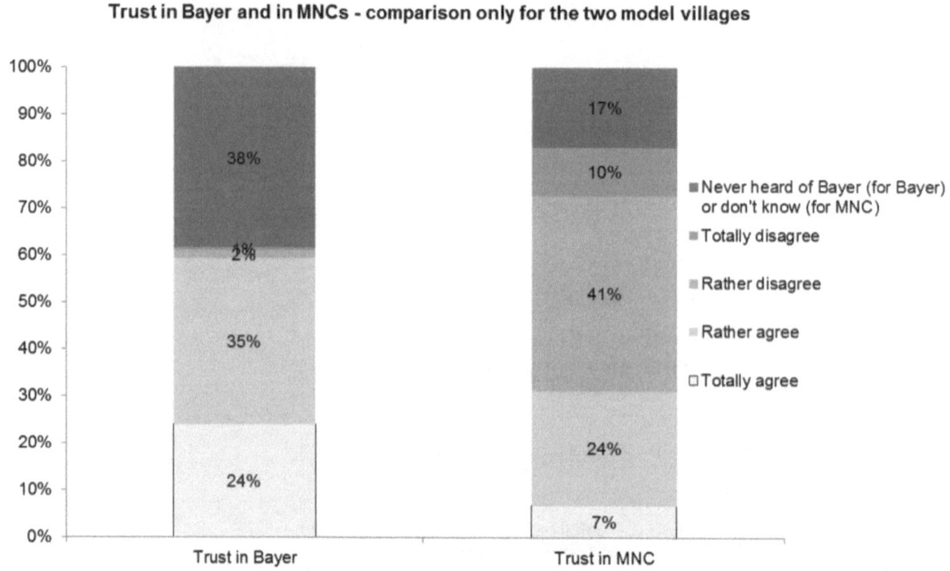

Figure 3. Trust in the model villages: Bayer versus Multinational Companies in general. *Questions*: What do you think about the following statements: I trust Bayer; I trust large foreign companies. *Source:* Model Village Project Survey, 2014, $N = 1190$.

However, any company will be restricted in this respect. Companies can provide instrumental freedoms (e.g. social opportunities), but they still depend on the people, specifically in terms of whether they are able and willing to convert their access to information and health care into valuable beings and doings. For example, parents and children decide whether they want to learn more about dental issues in dental health camps, whether the children attend the camps, and, most importantly, whether they are prepared to change their behavior. Dental health camps will have very limited impact if schoolchildren continue with their habit of chewing tobacco, which is sweetened for children but nevertheless still destroys their teeth. Hence, this example illustrates what Ruger (2010, 286) already described for health care: "Different people will convert the same access to health care into different health achievements and freedoms." However, besides depending on the people themselves, any company's efforts will also be restricted by the need to focus on business cases and competitiveness. Therefore, there is no real incentive for companies to undertake remedies for severe health issues that have no or only very limited impacts on the productivity of the suppliers (e.g. engaging in the mitigation of domestic violence, which appears to be widespread in the households). Even if a distinct productivity impact is seen, a company will have to refrain from initiatives that may improve the health situation and productivity but at economically prohibitive costs. In these cases, a strategic corporate neglect has to be expected. This can cause disappointment among external stakeholders who expect a comprehensive corporate solution. However, the associated risk of loss of corporate trust can be mitigated by communicating also the limitations of corporate strategies.

Not only may corporate strategies remain ineffective due to these reasons. Even corporate violations of health capabilities may occur, particularly when a corporate business case challenges people's health. For instance, illiterate and inevitably less informed customers may not be able to safely apply products such as pesticides. For instance, it is estimated that every year, 3 million people are poisoned due to the use of pesticides, 355 000 of them die and 750 000 end up with chronic diseases. Most of these incidences occur in the developing world (Atreya et al. 2011, 53). Therefore, an overall assessment of corporate impacts on health capabilities in the MVP has to address such risks of violating people's health and severely hampering SHD. Systematic training and information on safe use and health issues of the products are essential for a win-win situation.

8. Conclusion

8.1. The MVP: Lessons Learned and Perspectives

As discussed in Section 2, the CA and HCP emphasize that capabilities, autonomy, self-determination, personal agency and health agency, along with empowerment, are decisive measurements for the real freedoms of people. In this context, health capabilities have a central role for these processes and outcomes.

In times of restricted public funding, the global private sector, notably companies, has been called on to contribute to health capabilities (Cameron and Eyeson 2012). Our analysis has shown that corporate strategies can be identified that may be profitable and at the same time induce improvements in the domains of well-being, which are highly valued by the people (e.g. water purification, health camps, etc.). Our case has also shown that companies may even have incentives to stimulate government programs that officials have failed to introduce (e.g. the Malaria initiative). The outcomes of these strategies are important in gaining trust among the citizens. This has also been the case in the MVP, and has been achieved by providing instrumental freedoms, particularly access to health care, awareness raising and information. We find that these activities have resulted in a higher self-perceived well-being of the villagers.

Further research will have to clarify how far these subjective perceptions of higher well-being correspond with objective changes in the health status of the villagers and whether they can really constitute a win-win strategy. In the same vein, it has to be left to future research to assess the sustainability of the MVP initiatives in a long-term business case.

Beyond well-being, enhancing agency and empowerment are key issues for SHD. Together with other relational capabilities (Renouard 2011), trust may develop over time with increased information and good experiences among business partners (Fischer 2013, 253). As such, it will have to be assessed whether the MVP activities have also empowered women and other disadvantaged villagers. Empowerment is the foundation of personal responsibility and is critical because individually responsible decisions (e.g. on lifestyles) can be even more important for health capabilities than the instrumental freedoms, such as access to health care, that companies can provide.

Assessing potentially positive corporate contributions is important but should not ignore the risks in corporate strategies to neglect substantial parts of the population due to a lack of business cases. This confirms Ruger's (2009) caveat that MNC will not be able to undertake population-wide contributions to health capabilities. Moreover, in some cases (conventional agriculture is a relevant one), existing business cases have to be evaluated to clarify and mitigate risks of violating health capabilities.

8.2. Consequences for the CA

Our case indicates that the people-centered CA is a fruitful instrument for identifying the perceptions of the villagers and their deprivation of health capabilities. Our findings show the importance of Ruger's differentiation between health capabilities and health preferences. The health capabilities of the villagers are quite weak because their health behavior seems to be mostly aligned with their health preferences. These preferences seem to be affected through culture, accepted customs, habits and traditions. In part, Sen's arguments mentioned above—ignorance, fixed food habits, or apathy—might play an important role. Hence, the villagers are not able to utilize their whole health capabilities also due to their own restrictions and behaviors.

Building on this, researchers may use the CA to find out what corporate initiatives are valuable for the people as well as for building trust and establishing a win-win situation. More research is required by the CA to assess the positive and negative corporate impacts on health capabilities.

As health capabilities are not restricted to health alone, but also entail agency issues, the CA should further develop in a way that allows for a differentiated impact analysis of people's agency. Corporate activities can improve many villagers' agency by providing awareness raising and expertise, which are major prerequisites to decide on health issues according to what one values and has reasons to value. Nonetheless, MNCs can also establish new power and knowledge asymmetries between a company and its supplier villagers. It depends on the individual and collective agency whether the net effect will result in more personal agency or in an even higher dependency of contract farmers on corporate goals and strategies. Today, the CA is not well equipped for such an analysis. To assess this important issue, more CA research has to be devoted to issues of collective agency, institutions (Esquith and Gifford Fred 2010), and power inequalities (Stewart 2011).

Acknowledgements

This article is an expanded version of the presentation "Corporate contributions to health—the case of Bayer CropScience from the capability approach perspective" held at the 14th HDCA Conference 2nd–5th September 2014, in Athens, Greece. The authors would like to thank the editors and the two anonymous referees for their valuable and very useful comments on an earlier version of this article.

Disclosure statement

No potential conflict of interest was reported by the authors.

Notes

1. Among the few exemptions are Lompo and Trani (2013), Renouard (2011) and Schölmerich (2013).
2. Despite the fact that the Indian government has planned to deliver health care predominantly through the public sector, due to budget restraints, today, more than 65% of health services are private. Over 70% of health spending is out-of-pocket. There is also a shortage of health personnel, especially in rural areas (Reddy and Raj 2014).
3. For detailed information about the background and aims of the MVP, see Volkert, Strotmann, and Moczadlo (2014, 5–8).
4. Following the recommendation of the WHO, a person is considered to be malnourished if his/her BMI—defined as weight in kg divided by squared height in meters—is lower than 18.5 (WHO 1995, 7).

References

Agulanna, F. T., A. E. Ikpi, V. O. Okoruwa, and V. O. Akinyosoye. 2013. "A Synergetic Linkage between Agricultural Productivity, Nutrition and Health." *African Journal of Biomedical Research* 16: 1–9.

Alkire, Sabina. 2010. "Instrumental Freedoms and Human Capabilities." In *Capabilities, Power, and Institutions. Towards a More Critical Development Ethics*, edited by Stephen L. Esquith and Gifford Fred, 18–32. Pennsylvania Park: The Pennsylvania State University Press.

Alkire, Sabina, and Maria E. Santos. 2014. "Measuring Acute Poverty in the Developing World: Robustness and Scope of the Multidimensional Poverty Index." *World Development* 59: 251–274. doi:10.1016/j.worlddev.2014.01.026

Anand, Sudhir. 2004. "Why Health Equity?" In *Public Health, Ethics, and Equity*, edited by Sudhir Anand, Fabienne Peter, and Amartya Sen, 15–20. Oxford: Oxford University Press.

Asenso-Okyere, Kwadwo, Catherine Chiang, Paul Thangata, Kwaw Andam, and Daniel Ayalew Mekonnen. 2011. "Understanding the Interaction between Farm Labor Productivity, And Health and Nutrition: A Survey of the Evidence." *Journal of Development and Agricultural Economics* 3 (3): 80–90. doi:10.2499/9780896295421

Atreya, Kishor, Bishal K. Sitaula, Fred H. Johnsen, and Roshan M. Bajracharya. 2011. "Continuing Issues in the Limitations of Pesticide Use in Developing Countries." *Journal of Agricultural & Environmental Ethics* 24 (1): 49–62. doi:10.1007/s10806-010-9243-9

Bayer, A. G. 2014. *Global Compact – the Corporate Initiative of the United Nations*. Accessed July 3, 2014, http://www.bayer.com/en/global-compact.aspx

Biggeri, Mario, and Andrea Ferrannini. 2014. "Opportunity Gap Analysis: Procedures and Methods for Applying the Capability Approach in Development Initiatives." *Journal of Human Development and Capabilities* 15 (1): 60–78. doi:10.1080/19452829.2013.837036

Blalock, Garrick, and Paul J. Gertler. 2008. "Welfare gains from Foreign Direct Investment through Technology Transfer to Local Suppliers." *Journal of International Economics* 74 (2): 402–421. doi:10.1016/j.jinteco.2007.05.011

Cameron, John, and Abena Eyeson. 2012. "Connecting Developments in Corporate Human Management Thinking to the Capability Approach as Used in International Development Research." *Management Revue* 23 (2): 173–190.

Clapham, Stephen E., Kenneth C. Meyer, Cam Caldwell, and Grove, B. Proctor, Jr. 2014. "Trustworthiness, Justice and the Mediating Lens." *Journal of Business and Behavioral Sciences Twentieth Anniversary Issue* 26 (1): 55–74.

Deininger, Klaus, and Yanyan Liu. 2013. "Economic and Social Impacts of an Innovative Self-Help Group Model in India." *World Development* 43: 149–163. doi:10.1016/j.worlddev.2012.09.019

Esquith, Stephen L., and Gifford Fred, eds. 2010. *Capabilities, Power, and Institutions. Towards a More Critical Development Ethics*. Pennsylvania Park: The Pennsylvania State University Press.

Fischer, Christian. 2013. "Trust and Communication in European Agri-Food Chains." *Supply Chain Management: An International Journal* 18 (2): 208–218. doi:10.1108/13598541311318836

Feldman, Candace H., Gary L. Darmstadt, Vishwajeet Kumar, and Jennifer P. Ruger. 2015. "Women's Political Participation and Health: A Health Capability Study in Rural India." *Journal of Health Politics, Policy and Law* 40 (1): 101–164. doi:10.1215/03616878-2854621

Fleurbaey, Marc. 2002. "Development, Capabilities, and Freedom." *Studies in Comparative International Development* 37 (2): 71–77. doi:10.1007/BF02686263

Halpern, David, Clive Bates, Geoff Mulgan, Stephen Aldridge, Greg Beales, and Adam Heathfield. 2004. "Personal Responsibility and Changing Behaviour: The State of Knowledge and Its Implications for Public Policy." Prime Minister's Strategy Unit, Strategy Unit, Admiralty Arch, The Mall, London SW1A 2WH. Accessed October 10, 2014, http://webarchive.nationalarchives.gov.uk/+/http:/www.cabinetoffice.gov.uk/media/cabinetoffice/strategy/assets/pr2.pdf.

Iršová, Zuzana, and Tomáš Havránek. 2013. "Determinants of Horizontal Spillovers from FDI: Evidence from a Large Meta-Analysis." *World Development* 42: 1–15. doi:10.1016/j.worlddev.2012.07.001

Leßmann, Ortrud. 2013. "Empirische Studien Zum Capability Ansatz auf der Grundlage von Befragungen – ein Überblick." In *Der Capability Approach und seine Anwendung*, edited by Gunter Graf, Elisabeth Kapferer, and Clemens Sedmak, 25–63. Wiesbaden: Springer Fachmedien Wiesbaden.

Lompo, Kevin, and Jean-Francois Trani. 2013. "Does Corporate Social Responsibility Contribute to Human Development in Developing Countries? Evidence from Nigeria." *Journal of Human Development and Capabilities* 14 (2): 241–265. doi:10.1080/19452829.2013.784727

Mayer, Roger C., James H. Davis, and F. D. Schoorman. 1995. "An Integrative Model of Organizational Trust." *The Academy of Management Review* 20 (3): 709–734.

Moczadlo, Regina, and Jürgen Volkert. 2012. "Wettbewerb und nachhaltige Entwicklung bei globalen Governancelücken." In *Zur Zukunft des Wettbewerbs: In memoriam Karl Brand (1923 – 2010) und Alfred E. Ott (1929 – 1994)*, edited by Harald Enke and Adolf Wagner, 275–296. Marburg: Metropolis-Verlag.

Ng, Nora Y., and Jennifer Prah Ruger. 2014. "Ethics and Social Value Judgments in Public Health." In *Encyclopedia of Health Economics*, Vol 1. edited by Anthony J. Culyer, 287–291. San Diego, CA: Elsevier.

Nriagu, Jerome O. 2011. "Fluorine: Human Health Risks." In *Encyclopedia of Environmental Health*, edited by Jerome O. Nriagu, 776–785. Amsterdam: Elsevier Science.

Pirson, Michael, and Deepak Malhotra. 2011. "Foundations of Organizational Trust. What Matters to Different Stakeholders?" *Organization Science* 22 (4): 1087–1104.

Reddy, Srinath, K., and Mathur, Manu, Raj. 2014. "Developing Public Health Infrastructure in India." In *Routledge Handbook of Global Public Health in Asia*, eited by Griffiths, Sian, M., Tang, Jin, Ling, and Yeoh, Eng, Tong, 68–73. London: Routledge.

Renouard, Cecile. 2011. "Corporate Social Responsibility, Utilitarianism, and the Capabilities Approach." *Journal of Business Ethics* 98 (1): 85–97. doi:10.1007/s10551-010-0536-8

Ruger, Jennifer. 1998. "Aristotelian Justice and Health Policy: Capability and Incapability Theorized Agreements." Harvard University PHD Dissertation.

Ruger, Jennifer Prah. 2003. "Health and Development." *Lancet* 362 (9385): 1092–7.

Ruger, Jennifer Prah. 2004. "Health and Social Justice." *Lancet* 364 (9439): 1075–80.

Ruger, Jennifer Prah. 2006a. "Health Capability and Justice: Toward a New Paradigm of Health Ethics." *Cornell Journal of Law and Public Policy* 15 (2): 101–87.

Ruger, Jennifer Prah. 2006b. "Toward a Theory of a Right to Health: Capability and incompletely Theorized Agreements." *Yale Journal of Law and the Humanities* 18 (2): 273–326.

Ruger, Jennifer Prah. 2007a. "Rethinking Equal Access: Agency, Quality and Norms." *Global Public Health* 2 (1): 78–96.

Ruger, Jennifer Prah. 2007b. "The Moral Foundations of Health Insurance." *Quarterly Journal of Medicine* 100 (1): 53–57.

Ruger, Jennifer Prah. 2008a. "Ethics in American Health 1: Ethical Approaches to Health Policy." *American Journal of Public Health* 98 (10): 1751–1756.

Ruger, Jennifer Prah. 2008b. "Ethics in American Health 2: An Ethical Framework for Health System Reform." *American Journal of Public Health* 98 (10): 1756–1763.

Ruger, Jennifer Prah. 2009. *Health and Social Justice*. Oxford: Oxford University Press.

Ruger, Jennifer Prah. 2010. "Health Capability: Conceptualization and Operationalization." *American Journal of Public Health* 100: 42–49.

Ruger, Jennifer Prah, Dean T. Jamison, David Bloom, and David Canning. 2012. "Health and the Economy." In *Global Health: Diseases, Programs, Systems, and Policies*, edited by Michael H. Merson, Robert E. Black, and Anne J. Mills, 3rd ed, 757–813. Burlington, MA: Jones & Bartlett Learning.

Ruger, Jennifer Prah, and Hak-Ju Kim. 2006. "Global Health Inequalities: An International Comparison." *Journal of Epidemiology and Community Health* 60 (11): 928–936.

Scherer, Andreas G., and Guido Palazzo. 2011. "The New Political Role of Business in a Globalized World: A Review of a New Perspective on CSR and its Implications for the Firm, Governance, and Democracy." *Journal of Management Studies* 48 (4): 899–931. doi:10.1111/j.1467-6486.2010.00950.x

Schölmerich, Maike J. 2013. "On the impact of Corporate Social Responsibility on Poverty in Cambodia in The Light of Sen's Capability Approach." *Asian Journal of Business Ethics* 2 (1): 1–33. doi:10.1007/s13520-012-0016-6

Schoorman, F. D., Roger C. Mayer, and James H. Davis. 2007. "An integrative Model of organizational Trust: Past, Present and Future." *Academy of Management Review* 32 (2): 344–54.

Sen, Amartya. 1981. "Ingredients of Famine Analysis: Availability and Entitlements." *Quarterly Journal of Economics* 96 (3): 433–64.

Sen, Amartya. 1992. *Inequality Reexamined*. New York, NY: Russell Sage Foundation; Harvard University Press.

Sen, Amartya. ([1999] 2000). *Development as Freedom*. New York, NY: Anchor Books.

Sen, Amartya. 2002. "Why Health Equity?" *Health Economics* 11 (8): 659–666. doi:10.1002/hec.762

Sen, Amartya. 2008. "Capability and Well-Being." In *The Philosophy of Economics: An Anthology*, edited by Daniel M. Hausman, 3rd ed, 270–293. New York, NY: Cambridge University Press.

Sen, Amartya. 2009. *The Idea of Justice*. London: Penguin.

Smeets, R. 2008. "Collecting the Pieces of the FDI Knowledge Spillovers Puzzle." *The World Bank Research Observer* 23 (2): 107–138.

Srinath, K., and Manu Raj Mathur. 2014. "Developing Public Health Infrastructure in India." In *Routledge Handbook of Global Public Health in Asia*, edited by Sian M. Griffiths, Jin Ling Tang, and Eng Tong Yeoh, 68–73. London: Routledge.

Stewart, Frances. 2011. "Inequality in Political Power: A Fundamental (and Overlooked) Dimension of Inequality." *European Journal of Development Research* 23 (4): 541–545. doi:10.1057/ejdr.2011.23

Subramanian, S. 2011. *Bayer CropScience in India: Value Driven Strategy*. London: Richard Ivey School of Business Foundation, University of Western Ontario.

UNDP (United Nations Development Programme). 2010. *The Real Wealth of Nations: Pathways to Human Development: Human Development Report 2010*. New York, NY: Palgrave Macmillan.

UN Millennium Project. 2005. *Investing in Development: A Practical Plan to Achieve the Millennium Development Goals*. London: Earthscan.

UN (United Nations). 1947. "Chronicle of the World Health Organization: Development and Constitution of the W. H.O." I 1–2. Accessed July 17, 2014. http://whqlibdoc.who.int/hist/official_records/constitution.pdf.

Vanneste, Bart S., Phanish Puranam, and Tobias Kretschmer. 2014. "Trust Over Time in Exchange Relationships. Meta-analysis and Theory." *Strategic Management Journal* 35 (12): 1891–1902.

Vellakkal, Sukumar, S. V. Subramanian, Christopher Millett, Sanjay Basu, David Stuckler, and Shah Ebrahim. 2013. "Socioeconomic Inequalities in Non-Communicable Diseases Prevalence in India: Disparities between Self-Reported Diagnoses and Standardized Measures." *PloS one* 8(7): e68219. doi:10.1371/journal.pone.0068219

Venkatapuram, Sridhar. 2011. *Health Justice: An Argument from the Capabilities Approach*. Cambridge, UK: Polity.

Volkert, Jürgen, Harald Strotmann, and Regina Moczadlo. 2014. "Sustainable Human Development: Corporate Challenges and Potentials – The Case of Bayer CropScience's Cotton Seed Production in Rural Karnataka (India)." UFZ Discussion Papers 5. Accessed July 3, 2014, http://www.econstor.eu/dspace/handle/10419/95934.

Walters, David, and Philip James. 2009. *Understanding the role of supply chains in influencing health and safety at work*. Accessed December 10, 2013 https://www.iosh.co.uk/~/media/Documents/Books%20and%20resources/Published%20research/Cardiff-Brookes_RR_Feb_10.ashx

WHO (World Health Organization). 1995. Physical Status: The Use and Interpretation of Anthropometry: Report of a WHO Expert Committee. WHO Technical Report Series 854. Geneva: World Health Organization.

WWAP (World Water Assessment Programme). 2012. *Managing Water Under Uncertainty and Risk*. 4 vols. The United Nations World Water Development Report 4 2. Paris: UNESCO.

India, Health Inequities, and a Fair Healthcare Provision: A Perspective from Health Capability

RHYDDHI CHAKRABORTY & CHHANDA CHAKRABORTI

ABSTRACT *In India, health inequality, rooted in structural elements of the public healthcare system, is a topic of much concern and discussion in research literature. However, very few articles have approached this persistent problem from a theoretical standpoint. This article addresses this gap by employing the social justice framework of the Health Capability Paradigm (HCP). After critically analyzing some features of the Indian healthcare system, the article argues that some public healthcare system features not only cause health inequalities, but more specifically cause inequities in central health capabilities to avoid escapable diseases and premature death. To address such inequities, the article argues from an HCP perspective that the Indian healthcare system should (a) revise the national health policy's underlying vision of health, (b) reshape its three-tiered public healthcare system to deliver healthcare services to all, and (c) focus on core HCP concepts such as shared health governance and shortfall inequality as guiding principles to provide universal health coverage to all.*

1. Introduction

Health inequalities based on biological differences—the gap in average life expectancy between women and men, for example—cannot reasonably be described as unfair. These inequalities are not preventable or remediable. However, health inequalities may also be socially constructed and can be "unnecessary, avoidable, unfair, and unjust" (Whitehead 1992). Such ethically unacceptable inequalities, caused by various social and economic factors (popularly known as social determinants of health or SDH), are termed health inequities (CSDH 2008). SDH may be external or internal to the healthcare system, but affect and determine the health of individuals and populations living under them. Examples of such external determinants of health include housing, education, race, caste, class, income, gender, and social exclusion. Internal healthcare system factors appear on both the supply and demand side of healthcare service delivery, and include, *inter alia*, human resources, funding, and the use of services (Balarajan, Selvaraj, and Subramanian 2011). This article about healthcare in India focuses on some of these internal factors.

In India, health inequity[1] is a harsh reality. Health inequities vary according to social and economic groups as well as across geographical regions (Baru and Bisht 2010). The Scheduled caste (Sc),[2] Scheduled tribe (ST), socially and educationally disadvantaged people (constitutionally known as other backward classes or OBC (GoI 1980)), and the rural populations of the poorest states such as Uttar Pradesh, Bihar, Chattisgarh, Manipur, and Assam are more at risk of poor health than other members of society (Baru and Bisht 2010; ET 2014; WB 2015). Thus, children of the Scheduled caste are at higher risk of having anemia than children of the other social groups (Vart, Jaglan, and Shafique 2015). The tribal child born in India reportedly has a 50 percentage higher risk of dying before age 5 than the children of nontribal groups (Baru and Bisht 2010). Members of the poorest quintile suffer under-five mortality (U5MR) three times higher than those in the richest income quintile (Baru et al. 2010, 49).

Numerous researchers claim that these health outcome variations result largely from differences in availability, accessibility, affordability, quality, and utilization of healthcare services (Baru and Bisht 2010; Balarajan, Selvaraj, and Subramanian 2011; Bhagwati and Panagariya 2013; Dreze and Sen 2013). Some further claim that in a country such as India, differential qualities of healthcare service delivery and the inequalities in health service availability, accessibility, utilization, and affordability influence overall health disparities across regions, states, and segments of the population (Minnery et al. 2013); or, more definitively, that these inequalities cause India's health inequities (Baru et al. 2010; Balarajan, Selvaraj, and Subramanian 2011).

Researchers, social scientists, healthcare experts, and health policy analysts prescribe wide-ranging recommendations to address these health inequities. These recommendations[3] include reformation of the whole healthcare sector (Dreze and Sen 2013), bringing healthcare services under a local and national regulatory body (Bhagwati and Panagariya 2013), and investments in primary care services, application of certain principles (Balarajan, Selvaraj, and Subramanian 2011). But even though comprehensive, these recommendations fall short because they lack an undergirding theoretical foundation.

To fill this gap, this article draws on the social justice framework of the Health Capability Paradigm (HCP). It argues that health inequities caused by the Indian healthcare system and service delivery are not only inequities in health outcomes. Rather, they are inequities in the capabilities to avoid escapable disease and premature death. To address such inequities, the article argues for a change in the underlying vision of health in Indian national health policy. In addition, this new vision requires reconsidering the three-tiered public health system and incorporating HCP principles like *shared health governance* and *shortfall inequality* into the Indian health architecture. Together, these reconsiderations will shape a just vision for healthcare policy reform and help restructure the healthcare system to address central health capability deficits.

This article begins by demonstrating how features of the public healthcare system contribute to inequities in the capability to avoid escapable diseases and premature death—the central health capabilities. The health system's most significant inequities occur at this central health capabilities level. It then turns to key HCP concepts for guidance in addressing these inequities. As the first application of the capability approach to health (Ruger 1998, 2003, 2004, 2006a, 2006b, 2006c), the HCP and its antecedents, developing the field of capabilities and health, offers the most attractive theoretical and empirical approach for such analysis. Finally, the article, grounded in the social justice theory of the HCP, puts forth recommendations for the required vision of health, changes in the three-tiered public health system, and steps to incorporate shared health governance and shortfall inequality in the Universal Health Coverage (UHC) scheme to bring about fair provision for all.

2. Indian Healthcare System, Health Inequities, and Inequity in Health Capability

Both *public* and *private* healthcare structures constitute the Indian healthcare system. Responsibility for the public sector lies with the Indian government, but the sector is divided into three levels: central, state, and village or *Panchayat* level. This government-funded system is a *three-tier system*, with primary, secondary, and tertiary tiers. The primary tier, which consists of the Sub-Center (SC)/Primary Health Center (PHC), addresses health problems of the rural population. The Community Health Center (CHC), sub divisional, and district hospitals form the second tier. Teaching hospitals and other specialized hospitals form the third and tertiary healthcare level (Baru et al. 2010, 50; Acharya 2012, 54–55; Agnihotri 2012, 6). Unfortunately, this system is deeply inadequate for India's teeming population. Public health sector expenditures are less than 4 percentage of GDP (UNDP 2014). As a result, many complain about unequal access; low quality of care, diagnostics, and infrastructure; and a shortage of healthcare resources. To address some of these issues, the National Rural Health Mission (NRHM) was launched in 2005 by the Government of India (GoI) (Baru et al. 2010, 56–57) but its performance has been questioned (Sharma 2009; WG 3 (1), GoI 2011a, 7).

Researchers charge that the crisis in healthcare service delivery actually lies in its "massive inadequacies" in government spending and its emphasis on private healthcare service delivery and private insurance schemes (Dreze and Sen 2013, 143–181). They also cite nutritional failure, long-standing neglect of childcare services, and the "mere absence of public discussion of such inadequacies" (Dreze and Sen 2013, Ibid.). As a solution, these scholars recommend a new commitment to UHC by refocusing on the first tier of healthcare service delivery—that is, on primary healthcare centers—to deliver timely care on a regular basis; more public involvement in health issues; enhanced democratic discussion of health and healthcare issues; and the application of lessons learned in other nations and states (Dreze and Sen 2013, 177–181). The emphasis on UHC and open public discussion are valuable. But this prescription neglects the collective responsibility necessary to secure fair provision of healthcare to all. Nor does it specify how exactly to renew focus on primary care centers. It also does not specify the standard of quality for primary care service delivery, and what is to be the underlying vision behind it.

Highlighting five key areas of the Indian healthcare systems needing reformation, another group of researchers argues that the crisis of Indian healthcare involves public health inadequacies, routine healthcare, hospitalization and outpatient surgeries, human resources, and overall oversight of the system (Bhagwati and Panagariya 2013, 177–188). To these researchers, a systematic and substantial national-level regulation of healthcare services using a bottom-up approach and a strong scientific foundation for analysis can reform the healthcare system (Bhagwati and Panagariya 2013, 177, 188). The value of this recommendation lies in its emphasis on a bottom-up strategy. However, a bottom-up approach opens up different kinds of needs (regional, socioeconomic, and medical), and this proposal does not explain how to prioritize and address these needs. Additionally, addressing many serious health system issues, especially equity issues, require not just scientific analysis but also ethical reasoning. Healthcare reform under this regulatory approach might also produce a "one size fits all" strategy, which could overlook the neediest and foster its own inequities. Nor does this approach recognize the need for theoretical grounding in a theoretical framework such as the HCP.

Other researchers cite imbalanced resource allocation, limited physical access to quality health services, high out-of-pocket (OOP) health expenditures, health spending inflation, and behavioral factors affecting the demand for appropriate health care (Balarajan, Selvaraj, and Subramanian 2011). They recommend measures such as equity metrics in monitoring, evaluation and strategic planning; investment in a rigorous knowledge-base of health systems research; more equity-focused deliberative decision-making in health reform; and redefinition of the specific responsibilities and accountabilities of the key actors (Balarajan, Selvaraj, and Subramanian 2011). The recommendations, particularly the latter two, are useful in highlighting the demand side of the healthcare system. However, their recommendations are strategic, without any strong theoretical foundation, and they lack provision for in-depth insight about where exactly inequity lies and why it demands redress.

Despite these gaps, these recommendations are indispensable for healthcare reform in India. But we also need moral insight, theoretical guidance to address the deep ethical issues involved. Specifically, we need an underlying vision of health grounded in a strong theoretical foundation (Ruger 1995) and incorporating key theoretical concepts in the UHC scheme (Ruger 2008).

The following section explains how some features of the Indian healthcare system cause inequities in central health capabilities.

2.1. Some Factors of Healthcare System and Health Inequities

(*a*) *Healthcare Financing and Expenditure*: Public expenditures on health in India are low, less than 4 percentage of GDP (UNDP 2014). The private sector[4] has grown substantially, and its burgeoning growth is visible at all three levels (Agnihotri 2012). Findings of the last National Family Health Survey (NFHS)-3 (2005–2006) show that, due to public sector inadequacies, the private sector is the primary source of health care for over 70 percentage of urban households and 63 percentage of rural households (MoHFW 2007)[4]. This is one of the main reasons why such a large number of people in India are forced to incur heavy OOP expenses for private medical services, both for in-patient and outpatient care (Jacob John et al. 2011). In 2011–2012, the share of OOP expenditures on healthcare as a proportion of total household monthly per capita expenditure was found to be 6.9 percentage in rural areas and 5.5 percentage in urban areas.

Hospitalizations, even in public hospitals in India, have led to catastrophic health expenditures, and over 63 million persons confront poverty every year due to healthcare costs alone (NHP (Draft) 2015, MoHFW, GoI 2014, 8). This burden has been especially true in rural regions, where about 70 percentage of the Indian population lives. Half of them live below the poverty line and face major access and affordability barriers for quality healthcare services. Some of the direct consequences of such high healthcare expenditures are (a) selling of the household's resources, (b) cutting the healthcare consumption of other family members, and (c) borrowing money from lenders and slipping into debt (Baru et al. 2010, 53–54). In short, low government healthcare spending and high private healthcare expenditures push some groups of people down the socioeconomic ladder, where they face more socioeconomic vulnerabilities. It also forces them to compromise on medical needs and to ration care for themselves and their families, thus further undermining their health.

This high healthcare spending also forces people to compromise on nutrition and makes them vulnerable to diseases and death that could otherwise be avoided. A GOI report shows that these accessibility barriers are related to a rise in poverty-related malnutrition among some people (11FYP, GoI 2008, Vol.2, 129; Baru et al. 2010, 56–57). Research has also found that especially marginalized groups, who lack access to and utilization of health care, have higher rates of malnutrition resulting in anemia, morbidity, and mortality (Chatterjee and Sheoran 2007, 8). And malnutrition also links to other killer diseases such as HIV/AIDS (11 FYP, GoI 2008, 129) and acute lower respiratory tract infections (Kumar and Quinn 2012). These exposures and susceptibilities could be avoided if these groups were spared high healthcare expenditures.

In sum, low government spending on the healthcare system and high out of pocket healthcare expenditures make some people more vulnerable, both socioeconomically and medically, thereby creating inequities in social conditions as well as in health. Unjust susceptibility to malnutrition-linked diseases, especially resulting from high out-of-pocket expenses, implies that low public spending on health care and high personal healthcare expenditures diminishes central health capabilities.

(*b*) *Hospital Allocation and Capacity*: India has a 20 percentage shortfall of Sub-Centers, 24 percentage for PHCs, and 37 percentage for CHCs, particularly in Bihar, Jharkhand, Madhya Pradesh, and Uttar Pradesh (12th FYP 2013, III: 5). As of the last district level household and facility survey (DLHS III 2007–2008), at the all-India level, 49,193 persons are served by a single PHC, while the norm is to serve 30,000 persons in plain areas and 20,000 persons in hilly or tribal areas. And in many major states of India such as Bihar, West Bengal, Uttar Pradesh, Haryana, and Chandigarh, more than 150,000 people are served by one CHC (DLHS III (2007–2008), IIPS 2010: 214). The secondary and tertiary level public hospitals are largely built in urban areas and developed states (Baru et al. 2010). And failure to develop public hospitals in proportion to population growth and health needs has fostered growth in the private and corporate hospital sectors. In particular, private tertiary care has grown in the southern states, urban metropolises, and other well-off regions (Baru et al. 2010; WG (2), GoI 2011b: 15). These inadequacies in the number of care centers at the primary level and hospitals at the secondary and tertiary levels imply inadequate provision of timely care and treatment.

In hospital capacity (hospital beds, child birth facilities, diagnostic facilities, availability of medicines, and healthcare staffs), India has a current public sector availability of one bed per 2012 persons available in 12,760 government hospitals, or approximately 0.5 beds per 1000 (Planning Commission 2011a, 186). The number of beds in government hospitals in urban areas is more than twice than in rural areas (Balarajan, Selvaraj, and Subramanian 2011). In addition to this variation, differences in the allocation of beds appear among the states. In 2008, there were an estimated 11,289 government hospitals with 494,510 beds, with marked regional variation ranging from 533 persons per government hospital bed in Arunachal Pradesh to 5494 persons per government hospital bed in Jharkhand (Balarajan, Selvaraj, and Subramanian 2011). This disparity in the allocation of beds implies severe difficulty for some in accessing appropriate and adequate care.

As to diagnostic and critical care units, some have alleged that most public hospitals and medical colleges in India either have no viral diagnostic facilities (Jacob John 2005), or no intensive care units or ventilators (Jacob John and Muliyil 2009). Moreover, most of the critical units have been created at the district level, that is, in the urban facilities, thereby ignoring rural health needs (Jacob John and Muliyil 2009). Critical care units in hospitals at all levels bolster the capacity to address public health emergencies such as *A* H1N1, annual epidemics of dengue, chikungunya, and malaria. They can also help people seek timely diagnosis and treatment, and can help avoid needless loss of life.

This differential distribution of healthcare centers, hospitals, and critical care facilities has caused access barriers to some groups and individuals across geographical locations and socioeconomic factors (Deogaonkar 2004) and has given rise to inequities, especially at the level of health-seeking behaviors—the ability to seek appropriate, adequate, and timely care and avoid disease and death.

(*c*) *Healthcare Human Resources*: Like the inadequacies of hospitals, there is a dearth of healthcare human resources in India. Though government reports discuss recruitment, statistics do not match reported numbers. A recent government report, for example, states that nearly 150,000 skilled persons joined the Public Health System in the last 6 years under NRHM. Of these, 41 percentage are ANMs (antenatal nurse and midwives, responsible for taking care of rural women's reproductive health), 20 percentage are staff nurses, and 14 percentage are medical officers including Allopathic and AYUSH doctors (the indigenous system of medical practice involving Ayurveda, Yoga and Naturopathy, Unani, Siddha and Homeopathy) (MoHFW, GoI 2011, 40). This report also states that since June 2010, 1334 Bachelor of Medicine, Bachelor of Surgery doctors, 2003 specialists, 4892 staff nurses, and 3079 AYUSH doctors were added into the system along with 14,711 ANMs at the rural Sub-Centers (MoHFW, GoI 2011, Ibid.). However, in reality, low public healthcare funding has resulted in staff shortages at hospitals as well as in healthcare centers, and there are complaints about low quality in care and diagnostic facilities, especially in rural areas. Low quality care hinders opportunities to be healthy, obstructs health functionings, and hampers the ability to pursue health goals that one values.

Researchers found that in 2010, 10 percentage of posts of doctors at the PHCs, 63 percentage of the specialist posts at the CHCs, 25 percentage of the nursing posts at PHCs and CHCs combined, 27 percentage pharmacist posts, and 50 percentage of laboratory technician posts were vacant (Yeravdekar, Yeravdekar, and Tutakne 2013). These PHCs and CHCs are located in rural regions; so these rural areas suffer most from these shortages (Balarajan, Selvaraj, and Subramanian 2011). These rural populations thus lack timely and appropriate care; adequate diagnosis and treatment; and sufficient information about health, disease, and potential medical consequences. Adequate health center staffing would significantly diminish these health threats.

Beside shortages in human resources and adequate service delivery, rural areas also suffer from ill-trained and ill-equipped personnel. A cross-sectional descriptive study carried out among 225 Accredited Social Health Activists (ASHAs) in the southern state of Karnataka, between June and July 2011 found that ASHAs were poorly equipped to identify obstetric complications or to help expectant mothers draw up birth preparedness plans. Ironically, these ASHAs are to act as a link between pregnant women and health facilities and are trained to foster participation in Janani Suraksha Yojana (JSY, a safe motherhood intervention scheme to reduce neonatal and maternal deaths), institutional delivery, and immunizations (MoHFW, GoI 2011). As part of the NRHM, they are also required to have a birth preparedness plan and make pregnant mothers aware of the danger signs of complications to initiate appropriate and timely referral to obstetric care (Kochukuttan, Ravindran, and Krishnan 2013). However, while more than 800,000 women have been trained and deployed as ASHAs at the village level, till 2011 only 690,000-plus had received proper drug kits (MoHFW, GoI 2011).

This shortage of healthcare personnel, especially the ill-equipped staffs, affects access to and use of appropriate care. It has also affected immunization status across regions and groups. While all-India immunization coverage is low (44 percentage), the coverage in the highest income quintile (71 percentage) is three times than in the lowest quintile (24.4 percentage). And there is a substantial gap in immunization coverage between the STs (31.3 percentage) and others (53.8 percentage) (Baru et al. 2010). These disparities in immunization due to staff shortages have led to differential health status and disparities in the capability to avoid many life-threatening diseases.

In sum, factors internal to the healthcare system affect some groups, differentiated by geography, class, and caste, more than other, often by depriving these groups of information about health and disease and of equal access to timely, appropriate, adequate diagnosis and treatment. These factors affect the individuals' or groups' actual and potential health. Consequently, the affected groups have different abilities to meet their health needs, to pursue the health and life goals they value, and to adjust to and overcome new situations. As a whole, these healthcare-related factors hinder individuals' ability to avoid preventable diseases and premature death and thus exacerbate health inequities.[5]

To address such inequities in central health capabilities, the Indian healthcare system should provide fairly for all. And that needs reform at a much deeper level, beyond the healthcare system. The social justice framework of the HCP provides the requisite foundational framework. The next section provides an overview of such a paradigm along with a discussion of health capability inequities arising from the healthcare system.

3. Health Capability: A Social Justice Theoretical Framework

"Health Capability," a social justice framework for the reform of healthcare systems, health policy, and public health policy (Ruger 1998, 2004, 2006a, 2009), has roots in, yet extends significantly beyond, the *capabilities approach*[6] as propounded by Sen (1984, 1992, 2004, 2009) and Nussbaum (1997, 2001, 2003). With its roots in capability theory, the HCP, as created by J.P. Ruger, conceives health capability as a person's ability to be healthy and assigns a special moral importance to health capability, which signifies more than simple physiological health. Ruger defines it as, "... the ability of individuals to achieve certain health functionings as well as the freedom to achieve those functionings" (2009, 81). Here health functions mean avoiding disease, deformity, malnutrition, and disability; and reaching normal life expectancy. Freedom is the freedom of choice to pursue these functions. And individuals are agents who value certain health and life goals. Ruger identifies the core health capabilities as the *capability to avoid preventable disease and premature death,* conditioned by social, economic, political, and other factors (Ruger 1998, 2009, 4). These central health capabilities, as Ruger maintains, are not directly observable and measurable (2009, 81), but their component parts—health functioning and health agency (Figure 1)–are. Health functioning is health status or health performance. Health functionings of any group or individuals, Ruger specifies, can be known from existing health indicators and health performance based on those indicators (Ruger 2009, 8, 81–83). Good health functionings require collective societal obligations to ensure and enable the conditions for all to be healthy.

Health agency, the other component of health capability, is the ability of the group or individual to pursue valuable health goals (Ruger 2009, 82). More specifically, health

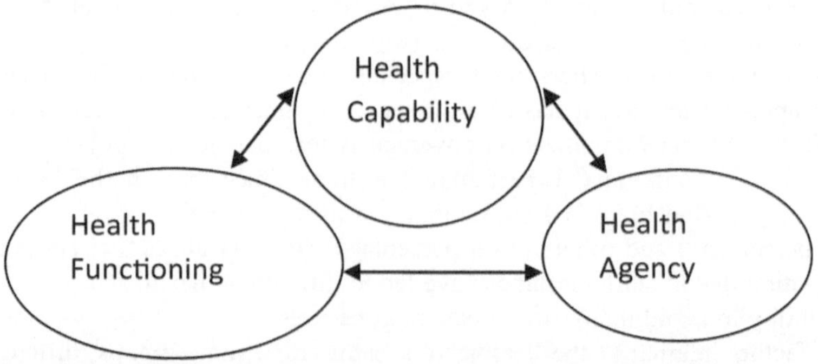

Figure 1. Health capability, health agency, health functioning.
Source: Ruger (2009, 82).

agency includes health knowledge, effective decision-making in health matters, self-management, and self-regulation skills (Ruger 2009, 146–148; 2010). And with health agency, Ruger incorporates individual responsibility for using healthcare and other societal resources and conditions to achieve maximal levels of health functioning. For, even if society guarantees equal access to healthcare, individuals must exercise their health agency to translate these resources into good health (Ruger 2009, 146–148).

Ruger claims that inadequacies in the healthcare system ultimately affect both central health capabilities and overall health capability. Therefore, according to Ruger, inequalities in health are actually inequalities in health capabilities and specifically in central health capabilities. These health inequalities prevent people from achieving good health.[7] She calls these deprivations "shortfall inequalities"; shortfalls of actual achievement from the optimal average. Ruger also suggests that these inequalities are social justice failures, *unjust* because they arbitrarily and unnecessarily reduce the capability for health functioning, and especially affect central health capabilities.

Because the healthcare system is a core determinant of health, Ruger further claims that health systems must offer individuals the prerequisites for a healthy life and positive health determinants. Those prerequisites within the healthcare system should be distributed equitably and should conform to high-quality standards effectively and efficiently. As part of the social justice obligation, society, through the government, should guarantee equal access to appropriate preventive measures and high-quality treatment.

She also argues that the public healthcare system and individuals have a shared obligation to create conditions where all can exercise health capability. She introduces the concept of "shared health governance," "a construct in which individuals, providers and institutions work together to empower individuals and create an environment enabling all to be healthy" (Ruger 2009, xiii; 2011). Shared health governance also requires universal health insurance coverage via shared costs and risk pooling, with health care funded through community-rating and progressive financing. It also argues for collective responsibility to enable equal access to high-quality care and expanded health agency by means of "reasoned consensus," a "joint scientific and deliberative process," and analyzing both clinical and economic factors for evidence-based decision-making (Ruger 2008, 1758). As a paradigm, the HCP proposes measuring the quality of healthcare by its ability to address functional impairments arising from injury or illness. And the impact of health care on individuals' health capability is assessed by examining health needs, health agency, and health norms (Ruger 2009). Health needs are directly observed through health functionings; health agency is judged through the shortfall of actual achievements from an agreed-upon optimum. Health norms are "societal norms about health that govern the environment in which individuals navigate choices for healthier life" (Ruger 2007). To address inequities in health capabilities, to help people to transform healthcare resources into optimal health functionings, these norms, Ruger suggests, need to be closely scrutinized, because norms can be either positive or negative and destructive.

According to the HCP, people become vulnerable and insecure when they lack access to necessary healthcare services. As a social justice framework, HCP focuses on vulnerability and insecurity. It is concerned with "individuals' exposure to risk and their ability to adequately manage it … " (Ruger 2006d).

Low public spending and high personal OOP healthcare expenses, as mentioned before, affect people's ability to avoid disease and premature death. In HCP terms, they adversely affect central health capabilities and cause inequities in health capability as a whole. OOP can actually restrict access to healthcare services, and thereby diminish the freedoms to pursue needed healthcare services (Ruger 2012). This barrier also impedes decision-making abilities and consequently affects health management abilities and health performance skills; that is, it affects health agency as well as health functionings. Besides directly hampering individual health agency and health functionings, it affects other related agencies. Thus, in the case of India, when OOP leads to cutting the healthcare consumption of other family members, it diminishes those persons' health agency. They then face deprivations in healthcare services and discrimination due to their ill health. And consequently, their health performances are undermined. Thus groups or individuals fall short from optimal health; they face deprivation in pursuing their health and life goals, and face increased risk of preventable disease and premature death. Thus occur shortfall inequalities in central health capabilities.

The lack of appropriate and effective distribution of resources, as mentioned before, leads to late identification and diagnosis of disease and inadequate protection for some groups or individuals. And consequently, those groups or individuals suffer more than others in the quality of care provided. In India, when distribution of healthcare centers, hospitals, diagnostic facilities, and critical care units varies by geographical location, it undermines some people's potential to avoid escapable disease and premature death.

A shortage of well-trained healthcare personnel not only hinder delivering quality and timely care, but also affects individual health agency and health performances. Ill-equipped and unskilled healthcare workers and the inefficiencies they cause prevent effective, efficient, and quality service delivery. And as a consequence, some individuals lack information about disease risks, health status, and how to protect against preventable disease and premature death. Similar inequities occur when a shortage of healthcare workers affects immunization and fails to cover all targeted people, as happens in India. As a whole, these shortages create inequities in health capabilities by affecting health agency, health status, and central health capabilities among groups.

Though it seems that the factors affecting the accessibility, availability, quality, and utilization of healthcare services are causing inequities in health outcomes or health functionings, in actuality, the inequities appear at much deeper level, at the level of central health capabilities. To address such inequities, reforming the healthcare system and service delivery in India must be based on a strong theoretical foundation of social justice. Having a strong theoretical foundation would help not just in strategizing the means to address such inequities, but also in developing a guiding vision to implement such strategies. Recommendations for addressing such inequities based on the HCP follow.

4. Recommendations

(*a*) *Health Policy and the Underlying Vision of Health*: To address inequities in central health capabilities and to enable a healthcare system to provide fairly for all, health policy in India should reconsider its underlying vision of health.[8] It is health policy that shapes and organizes a healthcare system. Viewing health as a capability and building upon the HCP as the foundational premise adds special moral importance to health itself and redresses inequities, keeping the variation in individual capabilities in view. Moreover, the goal of minimizing premature deaths and preventing escapable disease (i.e. ensuring central health capabilities) becomes a multi-sectoral action plan with the shared responsibility of different actors in individual and population health.

Health as a capability also emphasizes the importance of the individual in managing social, economic, environmental, and personal factors as part of health-seeking behavior. More specifically, it focuses on the individual's ability to adjust to, manage, and overcome risks and conditions created by disease and injury and affected by socioeconomic factors. And health as a capability also implies a capability to live up to average life expectancy. It indicates a potential to achieve an optimal average. In sum, health policy when grounded in the underlying vision of the HCP can shape a just healthcare system that accounts for individual and population health needs, health agency, health performance, and health norms. Viewing health as a capability in Indian national health policy grounds the reallocation of healthcare resources without any geographical or socioeconomic discrimination.

(*b*) *Reconsideration of The Three-Tier Public Healthcare System*: Though the Indian public healthcare system has been organized and functions at three different levels with the aim to deliver health to all, the system suffers from inadequacies, especially in funding and human resources. As a result, it fails to reach every individual, to deliver health to all, and to make a fair provision for all. This failure to reach every individual deprives some and creates inequities in health. In HCP terms, this lack of fair provision leads to inequities in the capability to avoid premature death and preventable disease. To address such inequities in health capabilities, the health system should reconsider its three-tier system and should try to deliver the highest attainable standard of health to all. Rather than having differential resources and infrastructure at primary, secondary, and tertiary levels, the healthcare system at the village, district and state level should be equipped adequately to provide high-quality care equally to all with increased government spending on health and the healthcare system. This implies, for instance, deploying critical care units, not just in all district hospitals, but also at the health center level, so that care is available at the primary level to avoid preventable disease and premature death.

(*c*) *Universal Healthcare Coverage and its Underlying Notion*: In India, the High Level Expert Group has defined UHC as follows:

> Ensuring equitable access for all Indian citizens in any part of the country, regardless of income level, social status, gender, caste or religion, to affordable, accountable and appropriate, assured quality health services (promotive, preventive, curative and rehabilitative) as well as services addressing wider determinants of health delivered to individuals and populations, with the Government being the guarantor and enabler, although not necessarily the only provider of health and related services. (Planning Commission 2011)

With this definition, UHC in India looks to provide opportunities, but does not accept full responsibility for the provision of equitable access. Moreover, with its focus only on "ensuring", UHC in India also overlooks the utilization abilities of individuals and groups. To address the inequities in central health capabilities and to provide healthcare service for all, UHC should both ensure and provide opportunities to achieve optimal health. When opportunities are provided, individuals and groups can exercise their fullest potential to pursue health and life goals. To do that, UHC should adhere to two core concepts of HCP, shortfall inequality and shared health governance. The shortfall inequality concept helps identify the neediest areas or populations and the gaps in service delivery. Shared health governance can guide the UHC scheme to shoulder the responsibility together with institutions, individuals, communities, and providers to "enhance individuals' health agency and create a social environment that enables all to be healthy" (Ruger 2008, 1751). These two concepts act as the guiding principles for identifying populations failing to reach target health status benchmarks, and for undertaking the collective responsibilities of ensuring and providing equitable healthcare access. The UHC should also adopt a "universal health insurance coverage via shared costs and risk pooling, with health care funded through community-rating and progressive financing" (Ruger 2008, 1757). With a community-rating, everybody pays equally, regardless of health status; progressive financing establishes higher tax rates for the wealthy to fund a functional health system (Ruger 2008). Continuous universal health insurance should protect "… all individuals at all times, regardless of changes in income, employment, or marital or health status" (Ruger 2008, 1758) from risk, both medical and financial, and enhance security and health capability" (Ruger 2006d).

In the Indian context, high OOP expenses prevent people from seeking medically necessary and appropriate healthcare services. Using HCP principles, the health system could bring all under the UHC umbrella and provide all with the opportunity to pursue good health.

To address high OOP, the Indian government in 2008 introduced a "national health insurance scheme" or "The Rashtriya Swasthya Bima Yojana" for people below the poverty line. Under this scheme, government pays the insurance premium; people are entitled to Rs 30,000 and may choose their healthcare institutions from the list of accredited health centers and hospitals (Dreze and Sen 2013, 152). While this is a step toward addressing healthcare-related inequities, HCP principles would require that this insurance scheme cover every citizen, rather than just some.

5. Conclusion

This article has sought to highlight sources of inequities in health capabilities in India. Addressing health inequities at the level of health outcomes only is naïve. National health policy should reconsider its underlying vision of health; the healthcare system in India should reconsider its three-tiered system, its conception of UHC to address pervasive inequities in central health capabilities. If it re-imagines health care according to HCP principles, the healthcare system can not only address the current unjust inequities in health capabilities, but can also provide health services fairly for all.

The social justice theory of the HCP (Ruger 2009) is the relevant foundation. The HCP introduces social justice to the health domain by drawing our attention to health inequities. Through core concepts such as *central health capabilities*, *shortfall inequalities,* and *shared health governance*, this foundational theory argues for collective social obligations, individual responsibility to use resources effectively and efficiently, and most importantly, for promoting health capabilities to raise persons and populations to benchmark goals of health achievement.

Acknowledgement

An earlier version of the paper entitled "Pandemic *A* H1N1 (2009) Preparedness Efforts, Compliance, and Some Ethical Considerations: A Retrospective Study on Hijli Rural Hospital (RH), Kharagpur I, West Bengal, India" was presented at the 12th World Congress of Bioethics held in Mexico City, June 25–28, 2014. Authors are thankful to the organizers of the conference for this opportunity. The authors are also thankful to the two anonymous reviewers and editors for their valuable insights and helpful comments.

Disclosure Statement

No potential conflict of interest was reported by the authors.

Notes

1. A historical review of Healthcare-related inequities in India revealed that three forms of inequities have dominated India's health sector; (a) historical inequities having roots in the policies and practices of British colonial India; (b) socio-economic inequities manifested in caste, class, and gender differentials; and (c) inequities in the availability, utilization, and affordability of health services (Baru et al. 2010).
2. Caste is one of the major socioeconomic determinants in India. Of the four castes, officially defined, Scs are lower in the hierarchy, largely rural and landless agricultural laborers. STs are the *adivasis* or tribals and face a similar kind of socioeconomic deprivation as the Scs (Baru et al. 2010, 49).
3. Space does not allow elaboration of the vast range of prescriptions here, and the recommendations stated here are also not exhaustive in nature.
4. The private sector accounts for 93 percentage of all hospitals, 64 percentage of all beds, 80–85 percentage of all doctors, 80 percentage of out-patients, and 57 percentage in-patients (Planning Commisssion 2011, 192).
5. In spite of these shortages, there are some notable success stories of prevention and eradication of some infectious diseases in India. For example, in 2012, WHO has officially declared India as polio-free. The success in this case has been attributed to a sustained and concerted effort, to an amalgamation of several factors, such as the very wide coverage of campaigns, improved surveillance among population, enhanced community monitoring status, and herd immunity. Most importantly, the success, as a whole, has been linked to the effort in identifying and addressing the gaps in the coverage on the basis of geographical location and of the socioeconomic background of the population groups (Chakraborty 2014).
6. The central claim of the capability approach is that assessment of justice and injustice should be in terms of each individual person's capability or freedom to achieve a level of functionings. It involves the individual exercising the choice to achieve a state of well-being. This approach conceives of creating the most conductive possible social conditions, i.e. arranging social, political and economic institutions so that adequate material and social resources are available to all, enabling them to possess and exercise a set of basic capabilities that help them lead a flourishing life (Alexander 2008).
7. Here Ruger adheres to the Aristotelian concept of human flourishing and health as the end of social and political activities. That is, good health involves participating in different social activities, being able to pursue further life goals.
8. In India, "health" has been conceived sometimes as a state of balance, as an adjustment with physical, social environment, as basis of economic development, as a constituent of quality of life, a complete state of physical, social, and mental well-being (GoI 1946:7, 1st FYP 1951–1956, GoI 2012: chp32, 6th FYP 1980–1985, GoI 2012: chp 22, 12th FYP 2012–2017, GoI 2013: 20.1), and as a right as in The National Health Bill Draft (MoHFW 2009). However, these definitions seem to recognize that economic development, but not total human development, is the only mark of a developed country. And "health" when considered merely as a right, it acts as an equalizer, rather capturing the diverse health needs of the population.

References

Acharya, Sanghamitra S. 2012. *Social Discrimination in Health Care Access, Among Dalit Children, Exploring Inclusive Environment*. New Delhi: Indian Institute of Dalit Studies.

Agnihotri, Anustubh. 2012. *Patterns of Regional Disparity in Health Outcomes in India*, Master Thesis, The University of Texas, Austin.

Alexander, John M. 2008. *Capabilities and Social justice, the Political Philosophy of Amartya Sen and Martha Nussbaum*. Farnham, Surrey, England: Ashgate Publishing Limited.

Balarajan, Yarlini, S. Selvaraj, and S. V. Subramanian. 2011. "Health Care and Equity in India." *Lancet* 377 (9764): 505–515.

Baru, Rama, A. Acharya, S. Acharya, A. K. Shiva Kumar, and K. Nagaraj. 2010. "Inequities in Access to Health Services in India: Caste, Class and Region." *Economic & Political Weekly* xlv (38): 49–58.

Baru, Rama V., and Ramila Bisht. 2010. *Health Service Inequities as Challenge to Health Security Oxfam India working Articles series. OIWPS–IV.* New Delhi: Oxfam India.

Bhagwati, Jagdish, and Arvind Panagariya. 2013. *Why Growth Matters, How Economic Growth in India Reduced Poverty and The Lessons For Other Developing Countries*. New York: Public Affairs.

Chakraborty, Rhyddhi. 2014. "Ethics in Pandemic Influenza Preparedness Plan: A Perspective from Social Justice." PhD Thesis, Indian Institute of Technology, Kharagpur.

Chatterjee, Chandrima, and Gunjan Sheoran. 2007. *Vulnerable Groups in India*. Mumbai: Centre for Enquiry into Health and Allied Themes.

Commission on Social Determinants of Health (CSDH).World Health Organization (WHO). 2008. *Closing the Gap in a Generation: Health Equity Through Action on the Social Determinants of Health. Final Report of the Commission on Social Determinants of Health.* Geneva: CSDH, World Health Organization.

Deogaonkar, Milind. 2004. "Socio-Economic Inequality and Its Effect on Health Care Delivery in India: Inequality and Health Care." *Electronic Journal of Sociology* 8 (1). ISSN: 11983655.

Dreze, Jean, and Amartya Sen. 2013. *An Uncertain Glory: India and its Contradictions.* London: Penguin Books.

Government of India (GoI). 1946. *Report of the Health Survey and Development Committee Survey.* Delhi: Manager of Publications, GoI.

Government of India (GoI). 1980. *Report on the First Backward Classes Commission. Vol I& II.* GoI. Accessed July 17, 2015 http://ncbc.nic.in/User_Panel/UserView.aspx?TypeID=1161.

International Institute for Population Sciences (IIPS). 2010. *District Level Household and Facility Survey,* (DLHS-III)*, 2007–08.* Mumbai, India: IIPS.

Jacob John, T. 2005. "Bird Flu: Public Health Implications for India." *Economic and Political Weekly* 40 (46): 4792–4795.

Jacob John, T., and Jayaprakash Muliyil. 2009. "Pandemic Influenza Exposes Gaps in India's Health System." *Indian Journal of Medical Research* 130: 101–104.

Jacob John, T., L. Dandona, V. P. Sharma, and M. Kakkar. 2011. "India: Towards Universal Health Coverage 1, Continuing Challenge of Infectious Diseases in India." *Lancet* 377: 252–269.

Kochukuttan, Smitha, T. K. Sundari Ravindran, and Suneeta Krishnan. 2013. "Evaluating Birth Preparedness and Pregnancy Complications Readiness Knowledge and Skills of Accredited Social Health Activists in India." *International Journal of MCH and AIDS* 2 (1): 121–128.

Kumar, Supriya, and Sandra C. Quinn. 2012. "Existing Health Inequalities in India: Informing Preparedness Planning for an Influenza Pandemic." *Health Policy and Planning* 27 (6): 516–526.

Ministry of Health and Family Welfare (MoHFW). Govt. of India (GoI). 2007. *The National Family Health Survey (2005–2006).* Vol. 1 and Vol. 2. Mumbai: International Institute of Population Sciences. Accessed August 1, 2014 http://dhsprogram.com/pubs/pdf/FRIND3/FRIND3-Vol1AndVol2.pdf.

Ministry of Health and Family Welfare (MoHFW). 2009. *The National Health Bill, 2009 (Draft).* New Delhi: MoHFW. Accessed March 11, 2014 www.mohfw.nic.in/nrhm/Draft_Health_Bill/.../Draft_National_Bill.

Ministry of Health and Family Welfare (MoHFW). Government of India (GoI). 2011. *Annual Report to the People on Health.* MoHFW, GoI.

Ministry of Health and Family Welfare (MoHFW). Government of India (GoI). 2014. *National Health Policy 2015 (Draft).* New Delhi: MoHFW. Accessed January 8, 2015 www.mohfw.nic.in.

Minnery, Mark, E. Jimenez-Soto, S. Firth, K. H. Nguyen, and A. Hodge. 2013. "Disparities in Child Mortality Trends in Two New States of India." *BMC Public Health* 13: 779.

Nussbaum, Martha C. 1997. "Capabilities and Human Rights." *Fordham Law Review* 66 (2): 273–300.

Nussbaum, Martha C. 2001. *Women and Human Development.* Cambridge, UK: Cambridge University Press.

Nussbaum, Martha C. 2003. "Capabilities as Fundamental Entitlements: Sen and Social justice." *Feminist Economics* 9: 33–59.

Planning Commission. Government of India (GoI). 2008. *11th Five Year Plan (2007–2012), Social Sector*, Vol. 2. New Delhi: Planning Commission, GoI.

Planning Commission. Government of India (GoI). 2011. *High Level Expert Group, Report on Universal Health Coverage.* New Delhi: Planning Commission, GoI.

Planning Commission. Government of India (GoI). 2011a. *Report of the Working Group on Disease Burden for the 12th Five Year Plan (WG 3–(1)): Communicable Diseases.* New Delhi: Planning Commission, GoI.

Planning Commission. Government of India (GoI). 2011b. *Report of the Working Group on Tertiary Care Institutions for the 12th Five Year Plan (2012–2017) (WG2): Tertiary Care Institutions.* New Delhi: Planning Commission, GoI.

Planning Commission. Government of India (GoI). 2012. *Five Year Plans.* Planning Commision, GoI. Accessed August 21, 2014 http://planningcommission.nic.in/plans/planrel/fiveyr/default.html.

Planning Commission. Government of India (GoI). 2013. *12th Five Year Plan (2012–2017), Social Sector.* Vol. III. New Delhi: Planning Commission, GoI.

Ruger, Jennifer Prah. 1995. *Health, Health Care and Incompletely Theorized Agreements.* Harvard University, Mimeograph.

Ruger, J. 1998. "Aristotelian Justice and Health Policy: Capability and Incapability Theorized Agreements." *Harvard University PhD Dissertation.*

Ruger, Jennifer Prah. 2003. "Health and Development." *Lancet* 362: 678.

Ruger, Jennifer Prah. 2004. "Health and Social Justice." *Lancet* 364: 1075–1080.

Ruger, Jennifer Prah. 2006a. "Health, Capability and Justice: Toward a New Paradigm of Health Ethics, Policy and Law." *Cornell Journal of Public Policy* 15 (2): 101–187.

Ruger, Jennifer Prah. 2006b. "Toward a theory of a Right to Health: Capability and Incompletely Theorized Agreements." *Yale Journal of Law and Humanities* 18(2): 273–326.

Ruger, Jennifer Prah. 2006c. "Ethics and Governance of Global Health Inequalities." *Journal of Epidemiology and Community Health* 60 (11): 998–1003.

Ruger, Jennifer Prah. 2006d. "The Moral Foundations of Health Insurance." *Quarterly Journal of Medicine*, doi:10.1093/qjmed/hcl130.

Ruger, Jennifer Prah. 2007. "Rethinking Equal Access: Agency, Quality, and Norms." *Global Public Health* 2 (1): 86–104.

Ruger, Jennifer Prah. 2008. "Ethics in American Health 2: Ethical Approaches to Health Policy." *American Journal of Public Health* 98 (10): 1756–1763.

Ruger, Jennifer Prah. 2009. *Health and Social Justice*. Oxford: Oxford University Press.

Ruger, Jennifer Prah. 2010. "Health Capability: Conceptualization and Operationalization." *American Journal of Public Health* 100 (1): 41–49.

Ruger, Jennifer Prah. 2011. "Shared Health Governance." *The American Journal of Bioethics* 11 (7): 32–45.

Ruger, Jennifer Prah. 2012. "An Alternative Framework for Analyzing Financial Protection in Health." *PLOS Medicine* 9 (8): e1001294.

Sen, Amartya. 1984. *The Living Standard*. Oxford Economic Papers, 36.

Sen, Amartya. 1992. *Inequality Reexamined*. New Delhi: Oxford University Press.

Sen, Amartya. 2004. "Why Health Equity?". In *Public Health, Ethics, and Equity*, edited by Sudhir Anand, Fabienne Peter, and Amartya Sen, 21–33. New Delhi: Oxford University Press.

Sen, Amartya. 2009. *The Idea of Justice*. Cambridge: The Belknap Press.

Sharma, Arun Kumar. 2009. "National Rural Health Mission: Time to Take Stock." *Indian Journal of Community Medicine* 34 (3): 175–182.

The Economic Times (ET). PTI. July 8, 2014. *Chhattisgarh highest incidence of poverty: C Rangarajan panel. PTI.* Accessed July 8, 2015. http://articles.economictimes.indiatimes.com/2014-07-08/news/51191636_1_poverty-line-least-proportion-tendulkar-committee.

United Nations Development Programme (UNDP). 2014. *Human Development Report 2014 Sustaining Human Progress: Reducing Vulnerabilities and Building Resilience*. New York: UNDP.

Vart, Priya, Ajay Jaglan, and Kashif Shafique. 2015. "Caste-based Social Inequalities and Childhood Anemia in India: Results from the National Family Health Survey (NFHS) 2005–2006." *BMC Public Health* 15: 537. doi:10.1186/s12889-015-1881-4.

Whitehead, Margaret. 1992. "The Concepts and Principles of Equity in Health." *International Journal of Health Service* 22: 429–445.

World Bank. 2015. *India Overview*. Accessed July 8, 2015 http://www.worldbank.org/en/country/india/overview#1 .

Yeravdekar, Rajiv, V. R. Yeravdekar, M. A. Tutakne, N. P. Bhatia, and M. Tambe. 2013. "Strengthening of Primary Health Care: Key to Deliver Inclusive Health Care." *Indian Journal of Public Health* 57 (2): 59–64.

Health Economics and Ethics and the Health Capability Paradigm

JENNIFER PRAH RUGER

ABSTRACT *Kenneth Arrow's seminal 1963 article "Uncertainty and the Welfare Economics of Medical Care," published in the* American Economic Review, *is widely regarded as the origin of health economics. The health economics field that has emerged in the subsequent 50 years has become a collection of market-based (demand for and supply of health goods and services) and non-market-based subjects. Despite a "broadening" of health economics to absorb ideas from other disciplines, the field has failed to pay adequate attention to ethics. Kenneth Arrow himself has called for greater attention to ethics in solving persistent health and health care problems for which economic tools are insufficient. The health capability paradigm is an attempt to integrate economic and ethical principles in an alternative analytical framework, enriching both health economics and ethics simultaneously. Social problems in health are so intractable that we must apply theoretical and empirical methods in both economics and ethics to analyse them. Health capability economics, as embodied in the health capability paradigm, offers a way forward.*

Introduction

In his *American Economic Review* article, "Uncertainty and the Welfare Economics of Medical Care," Arrow (1963) argued that medical care differs from other topics in economics largely because of the uncertainty inherent in disease incidence and treatment efficacy. Medical care does not fit with the competitive model of supply and demand, which is foundational in economics for its descriptive value and its efficiency in allocating resources.

The First Optimality Theorem of economics asserts that an equilibrium reached through the competitive forces of commodities priced in the market is optimal because no other equilibrium will make all market participants better off. The pareto optimality principle —there is an equilibrium state in which no one can be made better off in utility or other welfare measures without making another person worse off—is a value judgment, not a positive assessment. Pareto optimality is the end goal of social achievement, and this objective defines sub-optimality. The interpersonal comparisons on which optimality assessments rest come from the competitive market in participants' willingness-to-accept (WTA) and willingness-to-pay (WTP), with prices as signalling devices. WTA and WTP depend, of course, on initial purchasing power, conceived as asset and skill ownership. Transferring purchasing power from the well to the sick, for example through health insurance, increases the demand for medical care and thus the price as well.

Several decades later, Greenwald and Stiglitz (1986) proved that when there are asymmetries in information—adverse selection, moral hazard, or incomplete markets, all of which obtain in health care markets—then the economy is not efficient or pareto optimal. Actors do not take information costs into account, and there are interventions that can make some better off without making others worse off. Stiglitz continues to argue that there is no intellectual foundation, either theoretical or empirical, for the claim that economics requires getting markets right in health care (1991). Akerlof (1970) argued adverse selection is present in health insurance markets.

Rather Stiglitz (1989, 2012) asserts a strong role for government and believes the key question is how to design an appropriate set of health and health care institutions. He criticizes the US health care system because it is so inefficient and gets so little return on investment in contrast to other countries, a deficiency that cannot be explained by adverse selection (only sick people have come to America) or other deleterious American geographical or environmental conditions (Stiglitz 2012). Inefficient firms and institutions persist in health care and health insurance markets, contrary to standard economic theory predictions. Price distortions and rent seeking are major problems in a system with pervasive information asymmetries, and Stiglitz scorns public institutions for failing to address them (2012, 2013). Rather than assume market efficiency, Stiglitz argues, we need to start with the assumption that markets are not efficient, which fundamentally changes the analysis (2012).

Scholars have identified many other market failures in health, including imperfect competition (existence of oligopolies and monopolies, such as a few US insurance companies), failure to provide public goods (whose consumption by one person does not preclude consumption by another, such as medical information), non-marketability of health (health is not exchanged between consumers), lack of independence between supply and demand of health care, externalities, increasing returns to scale, and consumer irrationality.

Arrow (2012) has continued to argue that economic principles alone do not provide solutions to these and other health and health care problems, but that ethics and culture are necessary sources for principles to inform solutions. He argues that health and medicine are prone to "moral judgment" on multiple fronts. In the health care profession, an ethical sense of responsibility must guide conduct, rather than prices; traditional economic tools such as incentives for providers and consumers simply do not work. In society at large, where people's health is in the "public interest" and should be publicly financed, Arrow argues, insurance markets fall short. Ethical judgment is necessary because health care is not just a private good. Meeting people's needs requires developing a culture of ethics, accountability and efficiency in health and medicine (Arrow 2012).

Arguments from Arrow, health economics' founding father, might suffice to justify a greater integration of ethics and economics in health, but he is not alone in arguing for ethical principles in solving health economics problems. Stiglitz and Amartya Sen agree. Moreover, two of the primary health economics textbooks, *The Economics of Health and Health Care* (Folland, Goodman, and Stano 2013) and *The Handbook of Health Economics* (Culyer and Newhouse 2000) recognize the importance of ethical theory in health and health care, one of which states, "understanding what health care distribution is equitable and choosing what health care needs should be met in a society depends on ethical theory" (Folland, Goodman, and Stano 2013, 385). At the same time, bioethics needs economic theory because we live in a world of scarce resources and "economic analysis is based on the premise that individuals must give up some of one resource in order to get some of another" (Folland, Goodman, and Stano 2013, 10). This economic principle of "opportunity costs" applies to health and health care and cost minimization and budget constraints affect every individual in every society. The economic concept of efficiency is a powerful idea and tool to aid society in understanding the underlying costs and benefits to various policy options. Moreover, production functions, involving several inputs, are important economic tools for health production. Thus, any systematic theory or framework of health must include both ethical and economic concepts and tools. This article analyses critical problems in economic theory and argues for an alternative theoretical framework, the health capability paradigm (HCP), which fundamentally differs in the type of reasoning it employs compared to traditional health economics approaches. This health capability economics, as embodied in the HCP, offers a way forward. In the HCP, central health capabilities are the capabilities to avoid premature death and escapable morbidity.

Economic Theory and Rational Behaviour[1]

Rational behaviour is foundational to mainline economic theory. Standard theory suggests that a rational decision has three qualities: internal consistency of choice, maximization of objectives, and pursuit of self-interest.

Internal Consistency of Choice and Transitivity

There are several important analytical distinctions in internal consistency of choice theory. Being consistent in choice involves a mathematical structure of preferences based on binary relations. In making the best choice among S and R, the maximal choice is the set of elements for which a better element does not exist. The axioms of choice include reflexivity, completeness, and transitivity. In a binary choice between X and Y, standard theory assumes that the binary relationship determines all information about the choice function. In the *Foundations of Economic Analysis*, Samuelson (1947) defined preference as the binary relation that underlies consistent choice; the binary relation of preference is revealed through the consistency of choices taken. Revealed preference, along with the preference and choice relationship, is a building block of economic analysis.

But linking choice to preference as a behavioural assumption has limitations for understanding human behaviour more broadly and is a flawed basis for health economics. Choices in health and health care, either individual or social, cannot be represented by a transitive binary relation but rather have proved to be intransitive and even indifferent (e.g. a woman prefers not to have an epidural before labour (ex ante), prefers an epidural during labour, but after delivery states she does not prefer an epidural during her next delivery (ex post) or simply cannot decide on an epidural until she starts to have contractions in her next pregnancy). Indifference and intransitivity are particularly prevalent in health situations because people do not necessarily know their tastes for different health care goods and services and different health states over time.

Choice functions also require contraction consistency (a chosen alternative, X, must continue to be chosen even if the set of possible options from which X is chosen contracts) and expansion consistency (a chosen alternative, X, must continue to be chosen even if the set of possible options from which X is chosen expands). In global and domestic public health, these conditions ignore context. Contraction consistency implies that if I choose to vaccinate 15% of the world's population when choosing vaccination policies for the world (a larger set) then I would also choose to vaccinate 15% of the world's population when choosing vaccination policies for the city of Philadelphia (a smaller set in which vaccinating 50% of Philadelphians is an option). It may make perfect sense to choose to vaccinate 50% of Philadelphians born if the goal is to reduce infant mortality in Philadelphia (instead of choosing to vaccinate 15% of the world's population of children) but not if the goal is to reduce infant mortality worldwide. Another example would be for a person not to choose to be vaccinated for typhoid (X) when choosing vaccinations for oneself generally as an American citizen and choosing to be vaccinated for typhoid (Y) when as an American travelling for the first time to China or India. In the first choice the rationale is that one is at low risk and the vaccine is unnecessary and costly, whereas in the second choice the vaccine is seen as a recommended precaution worth the costs. Vaccination policies are related to context and experience. Numerous other health care and public health choice examples can illustrate the problem with these conditions, which fail to account for external objectives, values, or norms—all of which matter for decision-making and are included in the health capability economics framework.

The internal consistency of choice axioms that undergird mainline economic theory and sub-disciplines like decision theory, social choice theory, and game theory, are internal and link to component parts of the choice function. In mainline economic theory, behaviour reveals preference and is taken as legitimate, without trying to understand why people make the choices they make. But even perfect consistency in choice behaviour does not necessarily constitute rationality if one extends rationality to include external criteria such as norms and values. Numerous examples from the empirical literature suggest consistency requirements do not illuminate actual behaviour in the real word, thus reducing their descriptive and predictive reliability and validity and this narrow view's normative power. Rather, a rational choice should be viewed as having two conditions. The first, "correspondence rationality," is a necessary condition of a rational choice and refers to whether what "one tries to achieve and how one goes about it" (Sen 1987, 13) correspond. Correspondence rationality may be supplemented by "reflection rationality," that is "rationality requirements on the nature of the reflection regarding what one should want, value, or aim at" (14). This second condition depends on characteristics external to choice such as one's values, aims, principles and preferences, a wider set of motivations espoused by the health capability economics framework.

Self-interest Maximization

Standard theory also views rationality narrowly as self-interest maximization, excluding other ethical and social motivations, so much so that considerable work has tried to expand self-interest to include nearly all human motivation, even altruism. For instance, altruistic behaviour can be viewed as motivated only by the future reputational advantages or tit-for-tat payback it might secure. The predictive and descriptive reliability and validity of this view is problematic especially for cooperation amidst interdependencies, public interest, competing interests among individuals, and rules and codes of conduct. Nagel (1970) argues against those who deny the possibility of altruistic behaviour, asserting that basing one's actions only on one's own interests, and not those of others, is in fact irrational.

Self-interest maximization is primarily viewed as utility maximizing. "[A]ll human behavior," Gary Becker states, "can be viewed as involving participants who [1] maximize their utility [2] from a stable set of preferences and [3] accumulate an optimal amount of information and other inputs in a variety of markets" (1976, 14). In this way, utility links to revealed preference: when a person makes a choice, she is maximizing her utility, her self-interest or well-being. But other factors influence choice besides utility, self-interest or well-being (all representing her welfare). Kahneman, Slovic, and Tversky (1982) demonstrated that individuals frequently fail to systematically maximize their objectives, in research that has led to prospect theory and behavioural economics. Other lines of analysis reveal problems with the self-interest-maximizing view, including Schelling's (1984) bounded willpower (insufficient self-command or weakness of will), Simon's (1955) bounded rationality (individuals are not full maximizers), and the importance of institutions for human behaviour and social relations put forward by North (1981, 1990). These are important challenges to economic theory's foundations.

Sen (1985) has defined several elements that illuminate the concepts underlying these problems. He first defines self-centered welfare: here there are no externalities; my welfare only depends on my market basket, my own consumption, and I do not delight or suffer in another's market basket, well-being or actions. More formally: $W_i = f(C_i)$. Self-centered welfare is a fundamental property upon which major economic theorems rest. Self-centered welfare also excludes sympathy or antipathy towards others and concern for processes.

Sen's second definition is self-welfare goal. An individual's goal is to maximize her own welfare, or the expected value of her welfare under conditions of uncertainty. Others' welfare, actions or consumption are excluded. The goal function is expressed as $G_i = f(W_i)$ where the only thing a person is maximizing is her own welfare (W_i); or, if a person is including another person's welfare (W_j), $G_i = f(W_i, W_j)$.

The third is self-goal choice, a choice-making behaviour pattern exhibited by a person pursuing her own goals. A person's choices do not include the recognition of others' pursuits of their own goals.

While general equilibrium theory (Walras 1954) depends on all three elements—self-centered welfare, self-welfare goal and self-goal choice—the question arises: is it possible to violate one of these properties and not the other two? In health and health care the answer is yes. Take smoking, for example. Smoking violates self-centered welfare because it fails to consider externalities: smoking involves substantial externalities, especially associated with greater risk of illness for others from second-hand smoke and greater costs to society from tobacco-related health conditions and their treatments. But the person is maximizing her own (admittedly short-term) welfare, regardless of others' welfare or any codes of conduct about smoking, and is making the choice to smoke based entirely on pursuing her own goals (wanting to smoke). Personal goals can include other people's welfare, however, so if a person instead included others' welfare in her goal function, for example, $G_i = f(W_i, W_j)$, instead of $G_i = f(W_i)$, then smoking would violate the self-welfare goal. This example is critical for understanding the different policy implications of a standard economic approach (which defines a self-welfare goal as excluding the welfare of others) and a health capability economics approach, which bans smoking in public venues and allows government regulation of tobacco, recognizing other people's welfare as an important component of self-welfare.

Another health policy example concerns the pursuit of social justice. Motivated by justice principles, a person might embrace a goal of equal access to a basic health care benefits package for all people in her country. She might have health insurance herself and thus her stand has no direct bearing on her own welfare: the basic benefits package offered to others would not enhance her utility, well-being or happiness.

Similarly, a country might support universal coverage of a basic health care benefits package for citizens of another country unable to provide such services on its own. Of course, one can continually expand the self- and national-interest model to try to explain all individual or national behaviour by long-run self- or national interest. But this reasoning would exclude the range of values, norms, and priorities that do, in fact, motivate both individual and national action. For example, Norway's collective egalitarianism value might well explain its support for universal coverage in an impoverished country more accurately than some urge to enhance its national reputation or secure a tit-for-tat advantage. Health capability economics makes ethical reasoning central. Ethical motivations can be as powerful as selfish ones in determining both individual and collective behaviour, if not more so.

Game theory, in particular the Prisoner's Dilemma game, also illustrates the problems with the self-goal choice axiom. In this game, if each person follows self-goal choice, a strictly individual strategy regardless of what others do (the non-cooperative strategy), each person ends up in an inferior situation to the counterfactual, in which each would have followed a cooperative strategy. This result has held true repeatedly in studies, even when individuals follow their own moral goal-orderings but fail to take into account others' moral orderings. Important mechanism design findings in implementation theory (Maskin 1985) and incentive-compatibility (Myerson 1979), as well as the imposition of equity principles on social preferences (Fleurbaey 2007), offer insights for solving core problems.

The main problem with self-goal choice is that it fails to assess the implications of one person's own goals for another person's goals. Personal well-being, welfare and moral goal-orderings alone are not sufficient for optimal outcomes in multi-actor game situations. Rather, optimal outcomes require a meta-ranking of all possible rankings, including the rankings that consider self-goal and other-goal simultaneously. Violations of self-goal choice are relevant for normative and empirical reasoning in health.

In public health and health care, studies across the globe demonstrate people's ability to pursue their own health goals while also considering others' health goals, recognizing the mutual interdependence of everyone's health and health care benefits. For example, the largest insurance pool possible maximizes both the equity and efficiency of health insurance by distributing health benefits and costs among elderly, sick, young, and poor population segments and wealthy, healthy, middle-aged segments. In another example, the benefits of medical and health care research are so widespread that people recognize its value for their own goals as well as others', particularly those suffering from little-understood diseases whose diagnosis, prevention and treatment we seek to understand better. Supporting medical research might seem "irrational" from a rational choice perspective, but the social goals of this behaviour far outweigh the aggregation of individual self-goal choices across society. Self-interested maximization alone is an implausible behavioural foundation for health economic theory and policy analysis. An alternative view, based on a plurality of human motivations, is essential.

Utilitarianism, Agency and Freedom

Utilitarianism as the basis for social optimality has received extensive criticism. Utilitarianism has three elementary requirements: welfarism, sum-ranking, and consequentialism (Sen 1979). Welfarism involves judging states of affairs by the sets of utilities in those states; sum-ranking entails adding individual utilities as the correct method of aggregation; and consequentialism requires judging choices by their consequent state of affairs. Taking utility as the primary welfare metric means that utility reflects a person's well-being—but does it? An alternative understanding focuses on a person's agency, her ability to make commitments and form values and goals, and her well-being. One's agency need not focus entirely on her own self-interest.

Distinguishing between a person's agency and well-being aspects is important in understanding the behavioural foundations of modern health economics and ethics, but the utility-based welfarist approach does not make this distinction adequately, a health capability economics approach does. The choice literature often interprets utility or well-being as happiness, pleasure, desire fulfillment, and revealed preference. The well-being aspect, feeling happier or better off, may or may not relate to the agency aspect, the ability to pursue what one wants to achieve. Agency involves the ability to form objectives and to realize them. Desire is not a good indicator of health's value, especially in situations when one cannot reflect critically on one's health. For example, the effect of illness on health satisfaction is less in environments with more sick individuals, demonstrating that social health norm effects can influence self-assessed health (Powdthavee 2009; Thiel 2014). Moreover, the enormous variation in individuals' circumstances—the baselines for measuring incremental increases and decreases in well-being—makes utility an unreliable, insufficient measure of well-being. Even DALYs, an extra-welfare metric, are not equitable aggregate health measures (Anand and Hanson 1998). A better conception of well-being and a better and broader conception of the overall person encompass the capability to achieve valuable functionings, rejecting well-being as the only criterion for a person's welfare and utility as the measure of well-being. The well-being and agency of a person are more clearly seen in an individual's freedom, and two types of freedom in particular—process-oriented freedom and outcome-oriented freedom.

Health capability economics, as a framework of systematic theory, places freedom, not utility, as central. Freedom considerations, as opposed to merely welfare and utilitarianism, provide a framework for judging individual advantage and social optimality, equality and justice. A person's freedom is valuable in addition to her achievements. A person's opportunity or option for good health has value in addition to her health achievement. Four distinct categories are relevant for assessing the advantage or disadvantage of a person: well-being achievement, well-being freedom, agency achievement, and agency-freedom. This contrasts with mainstream health economics[2] which, even including extra-welfarism (Culyer 1989), takes freedom as being only instrumentally valuable and assumes individual agency is applied only to the pursuit of self-interest. But agency—and in HCP, health agency—have a greater role. Extra-welfarism has been advanced in health economics as a brand or adaptation of the capability approach, but it is not (Coast, Smith, and Lorgelly 2008; Hurley 2014). This mistake has led to inadvertent errors in reasoning such as the assumptions that the following constitute direct applications of Amartya Sen's ideas and the capability approach: including equity weights within the maximization framework, valuing process in utility terms ("process utility"), a focus on functionings exclusive of agency, and QALY's (a preference based health utility measure) as a capability metric (Cookson 2005). These efforts to move from welfarism to extra-welfarism in the health sector, while laudable, do not measure up to capability criteria and represent significant misunderstandings of what capability theory has to offer health economics.

Plurality, Incompleteness and Uncertainty

Moving past the limitations of economic theory's behavioural foundations reveals a variety and volume of ethical information that neither the standard health economic framework nor the extra-welfarist approach can accommodate. Health capability economics offers a fuller picture. Collapsing all relevant information into revealed preferences, utilities, happiness, monetary compensation (WTA or WTP) or achievement alone (e.g. health outcomes) and seeking complete or transitive ordering is insufficient. While health outcomes can give a partial view of health capabilities, a fuller picture requires health agency. Health functionings and health agency as objects of value are of different types and entail internal diversities as well. These issues of incommensurability and heterogeneity render complete and consistent overall orderings difficult if not impossible. Moving from the individual to the social level creates more diversity and plurality. Complete orderings and consistencies

—consistent and complete social welfare functions, requirements of economic theory—are unachievable, but partial orderings are possible. A complete ordering is not necessary to determine the best element in a choice set, so some incompleteness and inconsistency can be tolerated while making a partially justified optimal, if not maximal, choice.

This incomplete ordering applies especially when risk is uncertain and difficult to assess, as in many public health and medical care examples. Standard economic theory relies on expected utility as an approach to rational choice. Standard gamble methodology, which relies on probability assessments and expected utility calculations, forms the basis for health utilities, even extra-welfarist QALYs, in health economics. But uncertainty is a major problem in consumer rationality; sometimes probability distributions aid in assessing risk but in most cases both the probabilities and the necessary information about illness or treatment outcomes are unknown. Even predicting the outcome of a particular doctor visit or treatment regimen is difficult. Incompleteness and inconsistency are omnipresent in health and health care. People simply do not make the same health and health care decisions every time. In conceptualizing uncertainty, it is important to distinguish between (a) risk, uncertainty where probabilities are known (e.g. 50% chance of X, 20% chance of Y and 30% chance of Z) and (b) uncertainty, where we know that X, Y, and Z will occur but we do not know their probabilities. Knowing probabilities means knowing the frequency distribution of a particular event, the objective probabilities, whereas the subjective probability is the level of confidence one has in the occurrence of a particular event. According to economic theory if one is rational then one will follow Bayes rule, imposing an objective discipline of the frequency of events on the subjective assessment of what people themselves think will happen. If we know the frequency distribution of a given event A, then we know the risk of its occurrence; if we do not know the frequency distribution then we are uncertain about its occurrence.

The Ellsberg paradox tells us that presumed probabilities do not necessarily equal actual probabilities (Ellsberg 1961). It questions utility theory, which requires that people be equivalent between two lotteries in which the probabilities for one lottery are unknown. Expected utility theory requires that the expected value is $\sum_i P_i U_i$ where $\sum_i P_i < 1$ and $U_i \geq 0$. There is some circularity involved here when both probabilities and utilities are unknown such that probabilities are conditional on utility and utility is conditional on probabilities, hence a curvilinear relationship. The axioms of complete orderings, continuity, and strong independence are required and expected utility is determined by varying the probabilities among two lotteries, typically compounded lotteries, such that a person is indifferent between the two. These axioms fail to take process into account; expected utility is concerned only with outcomes and not process, a critique lodged by Broome (1991).

The Allais paradox is even more illuminating (Allais and Hagen 1979). In Situation 1, when given the choice between two elements A and A* where A is a lottery with 10% chance of $5 million, 89% chance of $1 million and 1% chance of 0 and A* is 100% of $1 million, people choose A* because of its certainty and the desire to avoid the possibility of 0. In Situation B, however, in a choice between B and B* where B is a lottery with 10% chance of $5 million and 90% chance of 0 and B* is a choice of 11% chance of $1 million and 89% chance of 0, people choose B. The paradox is that preferring A* to A violates the axioms of expected utility theory and in preferring B to B* the person contradicts herself. Allais argues that the paradox arises because utility theory axioms are mistaken in assuming that mental attitudes or magnitudes are the same in Situations 1 and 2 when in fact they are different. The situations must instead be understood as states of affairs, which include both the outcome and the process. Describing the state of affairs involves including mental magnitudes, well-being, processes and counterfactuals, what one could have gotten but did not get in a choice exercise. Fairness in process is not included within expected utility theory, a huge problem. But what are the alternatives? Prospect theory? Allais proposed another formula to expected utility theory, a polynomial formula, but the world is too complex and diverse to rely on a simple formula.

Ethical considerations are highly relevant for health economics but have not been adequately integrated in economic analysis; economic considerations are highly relevant for health ethics but have not adequately been integrated into ethical analysis. The failure to adequately take note of and integrate ethical considerations into health economics has left health economics weakened in its normative, descriptive and predictive abilities. A plural evaluative framework is necessary, and health capability economics and the HCP provides an opportunity.

Social and Ethical Motivations: The Common Good

A person might have reason to violate self-goal choice, depending on whether the unit of analysis is the individual, society, or both. If as a society, for example, we are trying to accomplish something together through partnerships then the correct unit of account is not just myself, but my group. Herd immunity in public health is an example. People create herd immunity together through individuals acting separately and getting vaccinations. Immunized individuals do not contract the targeted illness and thus do not infect others, thereby benefiting others. The costs of vaccination may be high, particularly if one includes time and lost productivity. Moreover, from a narrow rationality perspective, getting vaccinated may not seem like rational behaviour, especially for low-risk individuals. Yet individuals get vaccinated, to protect themselves, their families and their wider community circles. Individuals also voluntarily stay home from work or school so as not to spread germs. If everyone had a narrow view of rationality, not nearly as many people would get vaccinated, and herd immunity would suffer. Individual self-goal choices are suboptimal and inefficient from a social perspective. Voluntary other-regarding choice, in addition to self-regarding choice, enhances social optimality.

Individuals also reach decisions on ethical grounds. Much of our behaviour results from consciously rejecting some possible options because they simply are not the right thing to do. Under these circumstances, people do not change their objective functions, as standard economic theory would suggest, but rather they constrain themselves by reducing the possible choices. Kant's categorical imperative achieves this.

Rejecting the ethics-oriented view or social motivation view is unrealistic; ethics plays a role in actual decision-making. Other motivations include duty, loyalty, good will, following rules, value systems. Self-interest alone does not determine behaviour.

The Common Good

Collective action and cooperation are essential to create conditions of health. The individual's capacity for well-being links inextricably to the effective functioning of society; individual well-being requires an organized community that promotes the common good. Despite the axioms of standard economic theory, cooperation is not an anomaly but a hard-wired human characteristic. Cooperation, working together for common benefit, evolved in humans because societies that did not cooperate did not survive (Tomasello et al. 2012).

Empirical evidence demonstrates that cooperation requires fairness (Brosnan and de Waal 2014). Unfair situations generate negative responses; averting inequities advances cooperation. Institutional structures can foster such cooperation. These structures embody the interests of all, not a chosen few.

But why would actors cooperate? Why would they work together towards collective goals rather than continue to pursue self-interest? Even if actors did cooperate, why wouldn't they do so only in instrumental terms, viewing other actors as potential sources of costs or benefits as under a rational actor model (Ruger 2012)?

Extensive evidence helps answer these questions. There is abundant evidence of mutual cooperation and reciprocal altruism in humans (Dugatkin 1997) and of social motivations for effective cooperation—attitudes, shared identities, common values, trust in others' character and motivations, joint commitments, fair procedures, fair exercise of authority and decision-making, legitimacy, emotional connections—rather than narrow instrumental self-interest alone (Tyler 2010). We cannot be understood apart from our social context. Health capability economics recognizes these central elements (Ruger 2010).

Much scholarship focuses on socially and ethically motivated cooperation. Cooperation appeals to common identities, shared values, virtues, and a sense of obligation. Scholars contrast two motivational approaches, an instrumental approach of government rewards and punishments for behaviour, and a social motivation approach, socializing people into groups and supporting social ties. People are motivated to cooperate based on their own values and their links to social groups (Tomasello et al. 2012). Empirical studies in management, regulation, and governance demonstrate that social motivation is as effective as instrumental motivation, if not more so, because the increasingly collective activity requires cooperation, rather than compliance alone (Tyler 2010). Compliance requires significant resources to monitor populations and punish violators. In health, moreover, the goal is a healthy society with healthy individuals. People must willingly foster the health of their communities, their families and themselves, cooperation that legalistic rewards and punishments do not always or exclusively effectively motivate.

Inequity Aversion

Just as pro-social behaviour facilitates cooperation, anti-social behaviour—unfairness, inequities, a lack of trust, selfish acts and short-term self-interest maximization—undermines it. Experiment after experiment has found negative reactions to unequal outcomes like excessive over-compensation or under-compensation in games that treat joint contributions to a particular undertaking inequitably (Brosnan and de Waal 2014). Negative reactions include emotional responses (e.g. anger and moral disgust), rejection of outcomes and refusal to participate in cooperation, as shown in game experiments in many countries (Henrich et al. 2004).

Humans have evolved with a sense of justice and fairness, which facilitates cooperation, social reciprocity, conflict resolution, and shared endeavours. Research suggests that aversion to inequity is widespread in cooperative species under many conditions (including refusing immediately advantageous outcomes) and that it has evolutionary benefits. Humans experience both "first-order inequity aversion" (rejecting unfavourable unequal outcomes so as not to be taken advantage of) and "second-order inequity aversion" (rejecting unequal favourable outcomes) (Brosnan and de Waal 2014).

A central feature of the human sense of fairness is impartiality. We judge outcomes against an ideal, a standard, which applies to all individuals, not a chosen few. While humans differ by culture and circumstance, their common humanity provides the basis for core standards and ideals. Health economics needs impartial institutions that engender trust and legitimacy and seek to equalize states of affairs for all. Rational choice theory, standard economic theory, behavioural economics, and extra-welfarism offer limited guidance for effective health governance, health capability economics does.

The Health Capability Paradigm

The HCP (Ruger 1998, 2009) addresses many deficits in economic theory underlying current health economics. HCP does this by integrating economic and ethical reasoning for individual and collective health choices. While economic theory employs the ideas and tools of consumer theory, demand-and-supply equilibria and utility and indifference curve analysis, HCP uses a number of characteristic approaches to analysis. Distinctive features of the HCP, embodying health capability economics, include human flourishing and health capability; incompletely theorized agreements (ITAs); trans-positionality assessment; shortfall inequality analysis; production and cost modelling and efficiency evaluation; public moral norm considerations; procedural fairness; personal and social responsibility; and the study of uncertainty in the context of insecurity and vulnerability. HCP starts with an Aristotelian notion of the good life and societal goals of promoting good quality of life for all (Aristotle 1999). This view is broader than utility or welfare. It raises ethical questions relevant to economics, particularly health economics, since it helps us understand human motivation in both ethical and economic terms. Ethical considerations in health economics directly affect behaviour. Any framework of health economics must therefore incorporate them to provide more authentic normative guidance and descriptive and predictive explanatory power, if we are to enhance behaviour and find policy solutions to complex problems. Health ethics must have a central place in health economics, and long-held economic concepts and methods, such as technical and allocative efficiency and consequential analysis, must inform health ethics.

Most of the primary features of standard economic analysis, such as consumer theory and demand-and-supply equilibria and utility and indifference curve analysis, do not apply to health and health care. Behavioural economics and extra-welfarists moves, while laudable, tinker at the margins of a theoretical framework and tools that do not necessarily improve our understanding of health and health care. Rather than try to fit all the exceptions (e.g. to rationality from behavioural economics and to more than utility from extra-welfarism) to standard economic assumptions within the economic framework, an alternative framework that incorporates useful economic ideas and tools, for example on the production and cost side, within an overarching normative framework is likely a better prospect. Why? Because even welfare economics, behavioural economics and extra-welfarist economics, which themselves critique existing markets, rationality and health and health care distribution, do not provide the theoretical principles or positive analytical tools needed to understand the concepts of flourishing and efficiency that concern society the most. Inescapably, ethical theory is required to ascertain the reasoning and context to determine what society ought to do with respect to need and equity in health and health care, requiring a theory of health and social justice (Ruger 1998, 2004).

The HCP offers a set of values and criteria for assessing existing institutions and policies and proposals for reform. From a health capability perspective, justice requires legal, social, and political arrangements that enable individuals to be healthy. While the HCP is presented more fully elsewhere (Ruger 2009), in brief, HCP, embodying health capability economics, offers several unique resources for health economics and ethics and a way beyond the many current deficits in economic theory.

Human Flourishing and Health Capability

HCP is rooted in human flourishing, which values health intrinsically and more highly than solely instrumental social goods like income. It gives special moral importance to health capability, a person's ability to be healthy, which includes health functioning and health agency. It also recognizes that health underlies other types of functioning, including one's wider agency, or the ability to lead a life one values. Unlike standard economic theory, behavioural economics and extra-welfarism, health capability economics provides health agency to explain how individuals ought to and do behave about their and other's health. Restrictions on health agency have impacts on individual and societal health and well-being and the health capability economist seeks to better understand these relationships and devise policies to address them.

Social Choice Theory

A second unique HCP component relates to its theoretical and methodological approach to collective choice. The bioethics and public health ethics literature focuses sharply on democratic procedures for decision-making about health and health care. In espousing health capability as a substantive end, HCP addresses two important questions that standard economic theory, extra-welfarism and behavioural economics neglects: (1) how to obtain actual collective agreement on a dominance-partial ordering of health capabilities and (2) what type of social decision-making might apply.

This phase of the work draws on social choice theory and argues that ITAs form a complementary framework for the Aristotelian/capability view, providing a useful approach to collective decision-making in health and health policy (Ruger 1995, 1998). No unique view of health exists to evaluate health and social justice. The incomplete ordering of the capability approach, in combination with the ITA on that ordering, allows for reasoned public policy development and analysis amidst plural goods and different, even conflicting, views. Conditions of competition from standard economic theory and of maximizing the sum of consumer and producer surplus do not apply to health and thus the standard market equilibria where demand-and-supply curves intersect do not apply either. Yet the welfarist's and extra-welfarist's aggregation and maximization methodologies do not apply either rendering QALYs, WTP, WTA, Contingent Valuation inappropriate measures of health and well-being in collective decision-making.

Trans-positionality and Prioritization

This theory values "central" health capabilities above "secondary" ones. Central health capabilities are, simply, the capabilities to avoid premature death and escapable morbidity. These central features represent universally valued elements of health capability and offer a clear, grounded, and agreed-upon view. This model reflects an ITA on core dimensions of health capability. It provides a shared standard for health assessment. This view can help determine whether a particular public health or health care intervention or technology merits societal resources. Linear valuations, the cornerstone to welfare economic and extra-welfarist methodologies, as the summation of life quantity and quality components, do not bear out in the real world were people willingly sacrifice given QALY gains to prioritize critical health states such as providing resources for those who are severely ill. Central health capabilities have a special status that is not linearly superior to other non-central capabilities but that is important due to its vital role in human flourishing, prior to many other considerations.

Shortfall Equality

This view employs "shortfall equality" to judge public policies affecting health. Shortfall equality compares shortfalls of actual achievement from the optimal average (such as typical longevity or physical performance). The concept can also assess health capabilities, especially when equalizing achievements for different people is difficult. Human diversity is pervasive and consequential and can prevent some people from achieving maximal health. This approach is particularly relevant for assessing the health capabilities of people with disabilities because it accounts for differences in the maximal potential for health functioning without "leveling down" achievement goals of the entire group. This view also justifies having good health as an end goal of public and health policy even as we acknowledge that it is impossible to guarantee good health or equal health to everyone. Given the extensive deviations from the competitive model in health and health care, especially the assumptions under perfect competition, the role of uncertainty, information and externalities, and the normative pull of the notion of need in health and health care, need and need-based distributions are a central component of the HCP on a health capability economics view and a joint scientific and deliberative approach as below. In HCP health needs have a more independent and objective basis and health equity is conceptualized and measured in terms of shortfall inequality.

Public Moral Norms

Because health equity achievement requires resource redistribution, related legislation and regulation, and health-promoting individual and group behaviour, HCP requires an ethical commitment by all, those most fortunate and those in need, to health capability for everyone. Without this ethical commitment, redistributing resources from the wealthy to those less fortunate and from the well to the sick will not be possible, nor will health behaviour change. The effort to do so must be voluntary, that is, acts that are formed under fair conditions in which there is no duress or coercion. Individuals must embrace the public moral norm that health is worthy of social recognition, investment and regulation. The ethical imperative of health equity urges both individual and state action to help meet our own needs and those of others today and in the future. Standard economic analysis, extra-welfarism and behavioural economics provide no independent place for norms in their theory. In health capability economics, decision-making on ethical grounds is one idea behind individual and collective behaviour. Rational individuals making consumption choices under conditions of scarcity is not the main idea. Voluntary other-regarding choice in addition to self-regarding choice enhances social optimality in HCP. Unlike consumer equilibrium, a main idea behind HCP is the individual's capacity for well-being is linked to the effective functioning of society; individual well-being requires an organized community that promotes the common good; collective action and cooperation are essential to create conditions of health. Promoting the common good requires public moral norm internalization, a sense of justice and fairness as standards for cooperation rather than market competition.

Social Determinants of Health

How do social determinants of health fit within an overall bioethics or public health ethics theory? The "separate spheres of justice" view argues for focusing on justice in bioethics or public health ethics without reference to other public policy domains. Those who reject this view claim that bioethics or public health ethics cannot focus only on health, but must also address the many overlapping determinates affecting well-being. The HCP is more nuanced than these opposing perspectives. We are far from understanding the precise societal mechanisms influencing health, for example, the income and population heights relationship is "inconsistent and unreliable" (Deaton 2007, 13232) though clearly numerous policy domains impact health. It is reasonable to maintain the traditional criteria of a given policy domain affecting health (e.g. employment rates for employment policy) and to supplement those indicators with measurements of that domain's effect on health.

A Joint Scientific and Deliberative Approach

The HCP involves a joint scientific and deliberative process as a resource allocation framework. This public process combines the evidence base of health care and public health with input from individuals, physicians and public health experts to assess the value of treatments, medications and other interventions. It is important to assess both the necessity and the appropriateness of a health intervention. Although individuals have primary authority for health care decisions that affect them directly, physicians can help determine "medical appropriateness" and "medical necessity." In this framework, individuals employ their health agency, and physicians seek their patients' best interest. Physicians and public health experts share knowledge and resources with each other and with lay persons to balance technical and allocative rationality with ethical rationality; a more expansive account of rationality incorporates both. This approach incorporates participation and voice, but ultimately evaluates health policy by its effects on health capability.

Shared Health Governance

Decisions emerge from a shared concept of capability for health functioning. When disagreements occur, practical models of agreement or consensus yield workable solutions for standardizing prevention and treatment decisions and developing health policies and laws. This view contrasts with paradigms in which consumers alone, the market, physicians or public health experts alone, strict algorithms or cost-benefit calculations, fair procedures, or third parties, such as insurers, make health decisions. The underlying framework is shared health governance, a construct in which individuals, providers, and institutions work together to create an environment enabling all to be healthy. The decision-making of other approaches focuses narrowly on individual decisions in isolation based on rational choice, but a shared health governance model incorporates individuals' decisions for themselves and for their society. This paradigm promotes consensus on substantive principles and procedures of distribution, offers a method for achieving that consensus (ITAs), places importance on the results of health policies and laws (costs and effectiveness) in judging them, and promotes deliberation through collaborative problem-solving. Thus, the framework integrates both consequential (substantive) and procedural (democratic) elements of health economics and ethics. Neither the market equilibria of the standard economic model nor the social welfare function or maximal health of the welfare economic or extra-welfarist approach provide the basis for the allocation of societal resources because the basic assumptions of these models fail to approximate what is normatively attractive or how people actually behave.

Equal Access

Shared health governance approaches equal access differently. Equal access should mean equal access to high-quality care, not a "decent minimum," "adequate care," or "tiered health care." Equal access on this view does not imply equal outcomes or equal results. Nor is it enough to provide health care without efforts to expand individuals' health agency—their ability to navigate the health system and their environment to avoid mortality and morbidity and to meet health needs. Furthermore, shared health governance means shared responsibility—individuals, providers, and institutions have respective roles and responsibilities in achieving health goals. In policy terms, achieving equal access would require continuous efforts to standardize medicine, reduce medical errors, and move towards a gold standard of care. Such a view does not condone the significant disparities in health care quality that exist in many countries. Because both consumer theory and the social welfare function treat health and health care as one of multiple utility producing commodities, neither framework provides a valid and reliable basis for understanding societal choice in health and health care. Health need, rather than utility or price, provides a more objective and independent basis for assessing equal access to health care. Market outcomes are rejected on this view of equal access, health care need is the health care resources needed to achieve a threshold level of health functioning and health agency. In health capability economics, neither price nor utility are the basis for decision-making and professional ethics, rather than provider (doctor) self-interest, and health agency drive decision-making.

Responsibility and Health: Voluntary Risk

This theory seeks to enhance individual responsibility through improving health agency, as both are essential for achieving optimal health outcomes and creating a fairer health system for all. Any theory of health economics and ethics must address concerns of personal responsibility and voluntary risk. At first glance it appears that some people are not voluntarily averse to health consequences—smokers unconcerned about lung cancer, for instance. Some think people who knowingly take health risks should pay additional sums of money or be solely responsible for their health insurance and health care. However, understanding the causal determinants (including genetic determinants) of and differences between voluntary and involuntary contributors to health risk is difficult. Thus, blaming individuals for their health problems is often unjust (Wagstaff and Kanbur 2015). That said, improved health agency and health functioning can impose greater responsibility on individuals to make healthier choices and ultimately improve their health and the health of their community.

Moral Foundations of Health Insurance

A commitment to human flourishing opens up an alternative moral framework for analysing health insurance. Academic approaches to health insurance have typically adopted a neoclassical economic perspective, assuming that individuals make rational decisions to maximize their preferred outcomes and that businesses (including insurance companies) make rational decisions to maximize profits. In that approach, individuals who are risk averse will purchase health insurance. In empirical studies, however, individuals do not always make rational choices and consumer theory, the bedrock principle of standard health economics, is invalid, and neither extra-welfarism nor behavioural economics provide the tools for understanding the common bad of insecurity and vulnerability. Individuals also find it difficult to assess their health risks and to know how much insurance they need. Bioethics and public health ethics have focused on the issue of equal access to health care, but have provided little in the way of philosophical justification for risk management through health insurance per se. HCP argues that universal coverage is basic to human flourishing—to keep people healthy and to protect them from ill health's economic consequences. The HCP and health capability economics provides a more robust basis for understanding and analysing the role of health insurance, a major empirical reality in health and health care, for human behaviour.

Opportunity Costs and Efficiency

The HCP and health capability economics addresses a major void left in the bioethics and medical ethics fields; the crucial principle of opportunity costs and analysis of efficiency for health and health care. The HCP takes the idea of opportunity costs and efficiency analysis as essential, but it includes them differently from the standard economic model, welfare economics, extra-welfarism and behavioural economics. For example, these economic approaches entail reasoning at the margin, the costs and benefits of the next marginal unit are the basis for decision-makers (consumers, producers, or other entities such as government agencies) to make an appropriate choice. In this model, the incremental cost is traded off against the incremental benefit of a given service, product or investment. The realm of the coin is thus calculating and deciding optimally at the margin. The HCP and health capability economics is not wedded to marginal analysis in this way. Rather, this paradigm takes a step-wise approach to resource allocation whereby economic considerations follow and complement clinical input, not vice versa. Health capability economics, like mainstream, welfare, behavioural and extra-welfare economics, takes the scarcity of resources as a defining feature and major premise. Time is one of the many resources that are scarce. It is important to identify efficient programmes. Evaluation of health policies, laws, and technologies must consider costs because we live in a world of scarce resources. Moreover, every resource has an alternative use, so its expenditure corresponds with an opportunity cost. Therefore, some limits are necessary, and individuals and society, through shared health governance, must use these resources parsimoniously by evaluating efficiency. Cost-minimization analysis (CMA) and cost-effectiveness analysis (CEA) can be useful in comparing interventions for a single population, such as AIDS patients, by weighing the marginal benefits and marginal costs of two alternative interventions or different production possibilities. Both CMA and CEA are constrained by the ethical commitment to the ability to be healthy.

The consideration of costs under this theory resembles a utilitarian welfare economic perspective in that costs and outcomes are both valued. However, it contrasts with the utilitarian aggregation methodology and recommends CMA and CEA in combination with equity-oriented allocations (as opposed to incorporating equity weights into CEA). CMA and CEA can also reveal financial reasons for basic health care inequalities. Technical and allocative efficiency analysis can show opportunities for substitution of inputs and the best possible allocations for production to achieve health status goals.

Disabilities: Reasonable Accommodation

In societal decision-making about health care and public health, ethicists have struggled to address disabilities and severe physical and mental impairments. The HCP argues for basing judgments on joint patient–physician decision-making (at the policy and individual levels) and using medical necessity, medical appropriateness, and medical futility as criteria, rather than attempting to estimate specific weights for severely disabled individuals, as other frameworks do. It also rejects the marginal analysis of costs and benefits applied to disabled populations or disability categories allowable in the mainstream, welfare, behavioural and extra-welfare economic approaches. It does not, however, condone a "bottomless pit," whereby excessive investments in inputs have no or little effect on health capability, the diminishing returns to investment or production problem. Rather, costs should be considered, in a step-wise fashion, to ensure societal investments are made prudently. This may mean substitution or employing alternative techniques for health production that could more efficiently achieve health status goals. Thus, this paradigm aims to protect disabled people from discrimination while limiting exorbitantly costly care that would deprive others of health resources.

Conclusion

The HCP integrates consequentialist and deontological conceptions to determine the right and the good in health economics and ethics. It favours justice and health policies that, while not necessarily perfect or ideal, are "mutually acceptable to people whose preferences diverge" (Scanlon 1975, 668). To promote the good life, the HCP values core health capabilities—avoiding preventable disease and premature death—and favours those below the maximum average over those above it. It also emphasizes individual health agency and supports efforts to improve health for individuals so that they have the mental and physical capacity required for agency. The approach emphasizes shared decision-making at the policy and individual levels. This rational, evidence-based deliberative process involves individuals, physicians and public health experts. HCP offers a framework for integrating health economics and ethics.

Acknowledgements

An earlier version of this article was presented at the Human Development and Capabilities Association (HDCA) Annual Conference 2015, Georgetown University, Washington DC. I thank participants of the HDCA conference and the editor and two anonymous reviewers for helpful comments and Michael DiStefano and Francis Terpening for research and administrative assistance, respectively. I thank the Greenwall Foundation and the Catherine Weldon Donaghue Medical Foundation for support.

Disclosure Statement

No potential conflict of interest was reported by the author.

Notes

1. This section draws extensively on my notes from Economics 2057: Rational Choice, a fabulous graduate economics course at Harvard that I took with Amartya Sen in Fall 1995.
2. For definitive compilations of work in health economics see, Culyer and Newhouse (2000); Culyer (2014); Folland, Goodman, and Stano (2013).

References

Akerlof, George. 1970. "The Market for 'Lemons': Quality Uncertainty and the Market Mechanism." *The Quarterly Journal of Economics* 84 (3): 488–500.

Allais, Maurice, and Ole Hagen, eds. 1979. *Expected Utility Hypotheses and the Allais Paradox: Contemporary Discussions of the Decisions Under Uncertainty with Allais' Rejoinder.* Dordrecht: D. Reidel.

Anand, Sudhir, and K. Hanson. 1998. "DALYs: Efficiency Versus Equity." *World Development* 26 (2): 307–510.

Aristotle. 1999. *Nicomachean Ethics.* Translated by Terence Irwin. Indianapolis: Hackett.

Arrow, Kenneth J. 1963. "Uncertainty and Welfare Economics of Medical Care." *The American Economic Review* 53 (5): 941–973.

Arrow, Kenneth J. 2012. "Commentary on The Fifth Annual Kenneth J. Arrow Lecture: Moral Hazard in Health Insurance: Developments Since Arrow." Presentation at Columbia University, April 10.

Becker, Gary S. 1976. *The Economic Approach to Human Behavior.* Chicago: The University of Chicago Press.

Broome, John. 1991. *Weighing Goods.* Oxford: Blackwell.

Brosnan, Sarah F., and Frans B. M. de Waal. 2014. "Evolution of Responses to (Un)fairness." *Science* 346 (6207): 314–321.

Coast, J., Smith, R. D., and Lorgelly, P. 2008. "Welfarism, Extra-welfarism and Capability: The Spread of Ideas in Health Economics." *Social Science and Medicine* 67: 1190–1198. doi:10.1016/j.socscimed.2008.06.027.

Cookson, R. 2005. "QALYs and the Capability Approach." *Health Economics* 14: 817–829. doi:10.1002/hec.975.

Culyer, Anthony J. 1989. "The Normative Economics of Health Care Finance and Provision." *Oxford Review of Economic Policy* 5 (1): 34–58. doi:10.1093/oxrep/5.1.34.

Culyer, Anthony J. 2014. *Encyclopedia of Health Economics*. 1st Edition. Oxford: Elsevier.

Culyer, Anthony J., and Joseph P. Newhouse, eds. 2000. *Handbook of Health Economics*, Vol 1. Oxford: Elsevier.

Deaton, Angus. 2007. "Height, Health and Development." *PNAS* 104 (33): 13232–13237.

Dugatkin, Lee. 1997. *Cooperation Among Animals: An Evolutionary Perspective*. New York: Oxford University Press.

Ellsberg, Daniel. 1961. "Risk, Ambiguity and the Savage Axioms." *The Quarterly Journal of Economics* 75 (4): 643–669.

Fleurbaey, Marc. 2007. "Social Choice and Just Institutions: New Perspectives." *Economics and Philosophy* 23: 15–43.

Folland, Sherman, Allen C. Goodman, and Miron Stano, eds. 2013. *The Economics of Health and Health Care*, 7th ed. Upper Saddle River, NJ: Pearson Education.

Greenwald, B. C., and J. E. Stiglitz. 1986. "Externalities in Economics with Imperfect Information and Incomplete Market." *The Quarterly Journal of Economics* 101 (2): 229–264. doi:10.2307/1891114.

Henrich, Joseph, Robert Boyd, Samuel Bowles, Colin Camerer, Ernest Fehr, and Herbert Gintis, eds. 2004. *Foundations of Human Sociality: Economic Experiments and Ethnographic Evidence from Fifteen Small Scale Societies*. Oxford: Oxford University Press.

Hurley, J. 2014. "Welfarism and Extra-welfarism." *Encyclopedia of Health Economics* 3: 483–489.

Kahneman, Daniel, Paul Slovic, and Amos Tversky, eds. 1982. *Judgment Under Uncertainty: Heuristics and Biases*. Cambridge: Cambridge University Press.

Maskin, Eric. 1985. "The Theory of Implementation in Nash Equilibrium: A Survey." In *Social Goals and Social organization*, edited by L. Horasicz, D. Schmeidler, and H. Sonnenschein. Cambridge: Cambridge University Press.

Myerson, Roger. 1979. "Incentive Compatibility and the Bargaining Problem." *Econometrica* 47: 61–74.

Nagel, Thomas. 1970. *The Possibility of Altruism*. Princeton, NJ: Princeton University Press.

North, Douglass C. 1981. *Structure and Change in Economic History*. London: W. W. Norton.

North, Douglass C. 1990. *Institutions, Institutional Change and Economic Performance*. Cambridge: Cambridge University Press.

Powdthavee, Nattavudh. 2009. "Ill-health as a Household Norm: Evidence from Other People's Health Problems." *Social Science and Medicine* 68 (2): 251–259. doi:10.1016/j.socscimed.2008.11.015.

Ruger, Jennifer P. 1995. "Health, Health Care and Incompletely Theorized Agreements." Mimeograph, Harvard University.

Ruger, Jennifer P. 1998. "Aristotelian Justice and Health Policy: Capability and Incompletely Theorized Agreements." PhD thesis, Harvard University.

Ruger, Jennifer P. 2004. "Health and Social Justice." *Lancet* 364 (9439): 1075–1080.

Ruger, Jennifer P. 2009. *Health and Social Justice*. Oxford: Oxford University Press.

Ruger, Jennifer P. 2010. "Health Capability: Conceptualization and Operationalization." *American Journal of Public Health* 100 (1): 41–49.

Ruger, Jennifer P. 2012. "Global Health Governance as Shared Health Governance." *Journal of Epidemiology and Community Health* 66 (7): 653–661. doi:10.1136/jech.2009.101097.

Samuelson, Paul A. 1947. *Foundations of Economic Analysis*. Cambridge, MA: Harvard University Press.

Scanlon, Thomas M. 1975. "Preference and Urgency." *The Journal of Philosophy* 72 (19): 655–669.

Schelling, Thomas C. 1984. *Choice and Consequence: Perspectives of an Errant Economist*. Cambridge, MA: Harvard University Press.

Sen, Amartya. 1979. "Utilitarianism and Welfarism." *The Journal of Philosophy* 76 (9): 463–489. doi:10.2307/2025934.

Sen, Amartya. 1985. "Goals, Commitment, and Identity." *Journal of Law, Economics, and Organization* 1 (2): 341–355.

Sen, Amartya. 1987. *On Ethics and Economics*. Oxford: Blackwell.

Simon, Herbert A. 1955. "A Behavioral Model of Rational Choice." *The Quarterly Journal of Economics* 69 (1): 99–118. doi:10.2307/1884852.

Stiglitz, Joseph E. 1989. "On the Economic Role of the State." In *The Economic Role of the State*, edited by Arnold Herrtje, 12–85. Oxford: Basil Blackwell.

Stiglitz, Joseph E. 2012. "Commentary on The Fifth Annual Kenneth J. Arrow Lecture: Moral Hazard in Health Insurance: Developments Since Arrow." Presentation at Columbia University, April 10.

Stiglitz, Joseph E. 2013. *The Price of Inequality: How Today's Divided Society Endangers our Future*. New York: W.W. Norton.

Thiel, Lars. 2014. "Illness and Health Satisfaction: The Role of Relative Comparisons." SOEP papers on Multidisciplinary Panel Data Research: 1–43.

Tomasello, Michael, Alicia P. Melis, Claudio Tennie, Emily Wyman, and Esther Herrmann. 2012. "Two Key Steps in the Evolution of Human Cooperation: The Interdependence Hypothesis." *Current Anthropology* 53 (6): 673–692. doi:10.1086/668207.

Tyler, Tom R. 2010. *Why People Cooperate: The Role of Social Motivations*. Princeton, NJ: Princeton University Press.

Wagstaff, Adam and Rai Kanbur. 2015. "Inequality of Opportunity: The New Motherhood and Apple Pie?" *Health Economics* 24: 1243–1247.

Walras, Leon. 1954. *Elements of Pure Economics*. Translated by William Jaffé. Homewood, IL: Richard D. Iriwin.

Exploring Different Interpretations of the Capability Approach in a Health Care Context: Where Next?

PHILIP KINGHORN

ABSTRACT *In comparing the first applications of the capability approach (CA) to health and health care by Ruger with three subsequent interpretations of the CA, this paper identifies two distinct motivations: (i) the adoption of capability as an alternative to utilitarian health maximization, in the context of resource allocation and (ii) facilitating agreement on a core concept of health (incorporating mortality, morbidity and health agency) with which to drive policy reform. Where there is already comprehensive healthcare coverage, research is evolving to consider the broader impact of health on well-being and facilitate the joint evaluation of health and social care services. Although measures developed within this "expansionist" framework are becoming increasingly well used, their inclusion of health itself requires greater consideration. The health capability paradigm adopts health capability as a holistic object of health policy broadly conceived. Whilst instruments exist for assessing health functioning, qualitative studies are beginning to illuminate which indicators should be used to assess health agency. Shortfall sufficiency, a current pillar of the health capability paradigm, is considered as a potentially useful decision-rule when allocating health and social care resources. Setting a shortfall threshold will represent a value judgement and this should be informed through public deliberation and debate. The implications of adopting shortfall sufficiency also need to be explored and alternatives considered.*

Introduction

Given the scarcity of healthcare resources, it is deemed important to justify the provision (or indeed the withdrawal) of an intervention or programme based upon its value. Economic analysis aims to assess the value (the "goodness") of interventions and programmes through a systematic comparison of benefits and costs (Broome 2000). Approaches differ mainly in respect to how benefits are defined and assessed. One common form of economic evaluation used by health economists across many countries is cost–utility analysis,[1] and in turn, this is commonly operationalized using quality-adjusted life years (QALYs).

Within a strictly welfarist approach, utility is the (only) appropriate metric for assessing the goodness of different states of the world and it is individuals (consumers or households) who are the best judges of which state they would rather be in (Brouwer et al. 2008). The "extra-welfarist approach" (the approach within which QALYs are justified) relaxes the "undue information restriction" imposed by welfarism so that extra-welfare elements (i.e. non-utility aspects) are also embodied in the judgement of social states (Culyer 1991, 67). The extra-welfare element suggested for inclusion is health—health functioning and life expectancy. "Utility" is used as a means of ranking preferences or choices over different health-related quality of life states (Culyer 1991).

Utility weights for each health state are treated as cardinal values which lie on a scale that is established by assigning a value of 1 to being in full health and 0 to being dead (Torrance 1986). QALYs are then calculated by multiplying the utility weights reflecting the relative goodness of a health state by the amount of time spent in that health state, summing over all time periods and standardizing to a year (Morris, Devlin, and Parkin 2007). The value of a particular health state is judged from a societal perspective (through the aggregation of individual preferences, elicited using methods such as standard gamble and time trade-off), and a unit of "health" is assumed to be of equal value for all individuals (Culyer 1991, 53).

The QALY framework rests on the assertion that what matters to decision-makers and to society is the maximization of health. Even if the equity implications associated with health maximization are accepted, there is a need within extra-welfarist approaches to define health, or at least to collect data which give a reasonable proxy indication of patients' health status. Perhaps the best-known definition of health is that from the World Health Organisation:

> Health is a state of complete physical, mental and social well-being and not merely the absence of disease or infirmity. (WHO 1946, 100)

Generic multi-attribute health status classification systems such as the EQ-5D, SF-6D, and HUI are commonly used to assess health-related quality of life in practice and the focus on health functioning within these measures has led to comparisons with the capability approach (CA). Some authors have gone as far as to suggest reinterpreting the current QALY as a "cardinal and interpersonally comparable index of the value of the individual's capability set" (Cookson 2005, 818). Whilst Sen's work may have influenced advocates of extra-welfarism, it is more appropriate to think of the QALY (as it is currently operationalized) as a narrow practical and workable framework, developed within a specialist and policy-focused area of the economics discipline, rather than as anything more theoretically or normatively ambitious. Saith argues that, "extra-welfarism" falls short of what is proposed by the CA in at least three areas, namely, an exclusive focus on health, rather than multiple dimensions; a focus on health-related functionings as opposed to capabilities; and a focus on maximizing the gains in health rather than concerns with equity (Saith 2011, 590–591). Extra-welfarism also still relies on utilities and health preferences.

A number of authors have advocated use of the CA as an alternative to the QALY (Anand 2005; Coast, Smith, and Lorgelly 2008a; Coast, Smith, and Lorgelly 2008b; Ruger 1998; Ruger 2004a; Ruger 2009a; Verkerk, Busschbach, and Karssing 2001). But, what does the CA tell us about how scarce healthcare resources should be allocated, and how do we go about using the approach? Furthermore, are we able to operationalize capability in health without finding that we have reinvented the QALY?

Given that the underlying conceptual framework is incomplete (Robeyns 2006), seeking answers to these questions is challenging. It is largely left to the individual researcher to identify key principles from Sen's work and to build their application around these principles:

> the reader who looks for a fully formulated account of social justice ... in Sen's work will not find one; he or she will need to extrapolate one from the suggestive materials Sen provides. (Nussbaum 2003, 34)

The first applications of the CA to health and health care were put forward by Ruger (1998), beginning nearly 20 years ago, originating and defining the field of capabilities in this context. More specifically, to the question posed above, Ruger developed a framework for understanding how scarce resources should be allocated and provided guidance on how to go about using her approach (Ruger 1998, 2004a, 2009b). Since that time, differing interpretations of the CA have been published and will be outlined in this paper. It is of no surprise—given the underspecified nature of the underlying framework—that they differ significantly in several key respects. Having taken stock of the starting point and evolution of attempts to operationalize the CA in a health and healthcare context to date, beginning with Ruger's work, a possible path for future research will be suggested, along with the issues that will need to be addressed by those choosing to follow it.

Interpretations of the CA Relating to Health and Health Care

Four broad programmes of work will be introduced in this section and explored, in turn, according to: the methods used to select relevant capabilities and the scope of the capability set; valuation of the capabilities/choice of weightings; the decision-rule to be adopted (where specified).

Defining the Capability Set

Ruger's Health Capability Paradigm. In the first applications of the CA within the context of health and health care, Ruger's Health Capability Paradigm embodies an Aristotelian view of human flourishing and is concerned with the ability of individuals to realize two central health capabilities: the capability to avoid premature mortality and the capability to avoid premature morbidity (Ruger 2009b, 81). Alongside health functionings within the health capability paradigm is "health agency:" "the ability to acquire and draw on health-related information, knowledge, and skills to preserve health and develop a set of habits and conditions to prevent, to the extent possible, the onset of morbidity and mortality" (Ruger 2009b, 44).

The difficulty associated with defining and the lack of any unanimous account of health is acknowledged by Ruger. In selecting premature mortality and avoidable morbidity, Ruger aims to specify an objective global standard for assessing health. Ruger intends her conception of health to reflect the "view from everywhere" (Ruger 2009b). At an individual (internal) level, Ruger suggests that health status and health functioning could, but need not be, assessed using instruments such as SF-36 and according to life expectancy, child and infant mortality and the presence or absence of various biomarkers and diseases (Ruger 2004a; Ruger and Kim 2006). In order to evaluate the internal dimension of health policy in the health capability paradigm, one would therefore assess realized health functionings, using measures which, in most cases, already exist (Ruger 1998, 2004a, 2009b, 76). Used only as a proxy, these observed health functionings will offer a partial view of health capabilities (Ruger 2009a, 113), but it is stated that "health capabilities are not [themselves] directly observable" (Ruger 2009a, P79). Alongside health capability is the concept of health agency and hence health knowledge would also be promoted (e.g. the degree to which risk factors are explained, services signposted and individuals are able to make informed decisions about lifestyle and health goals). Affecting health capability and health agency are, at the external level, social norms, social networks and group membership and material circumstances; such influences would be assessed via the health capability profile specified by researchers and policy-makers employing the paradigm and profile. For example, the external (or social/cultural) level of the health capability paradigm has been adopted as a framework for empirically analysing and understanding the impact of health insurance reforms, with financial protection being assumed to reduce health vulnerability (Nguyen et al. 2012; Ruger 2012), the effect of health expenses on household capabilities and coping mechanisms among poor households (Nguyen et al. 2012) in Vietnam. Qualitative work has also explored the concept of health agency (Feldman et al. 2014).

OCAP/OxCAP instruments. Lorgelly et al. (2008) set out to refine an existing survey, composed of 60 indicators which, in turn, had originally been selected from the British Household Panel Survey by Anand, Hunter, and Smith (2005) on the basis that they related to Nussbaum's 10 central capabilities. Lorgelly et al. refined the list of 60 questions through 2 phases of participatory work, to arrive at an index of 18 questions (OCAP-18), related to capability, which can be used to evaluate complex public health interventions.

Some of the 18 questions are phrased in terms of functioning (such as "How suitable or unsuitable is your accommodation for your current needs?"), whereas others ask about ability (such as "Are you able to meet socially with friends, relatives and work colleagues?") and could be interpreted as capturing self-perceived capability.

Lorgelly et al.'s list of 18 capability-related questions have since been further adapted to form the OxCAP-MH, a capability-based questionnaire for use in the context of mental health (Simon et al. 2013). Again, the dimensions within the OxCAP-MH are phrased in terms of both functioning (for example, "does your health limit in any way your usual activities?") and capability (for example, "I am able to influence decisions affecting my local area").

ICECAP instruments. The ICECAP-O used purely participatory methods to define the capability set and affiliated questionnaire. The range of ICECAP instruments now includes: the ICECAP-O (for use with older people) (Grewal et al. 2006); ICECAP-A (for the general adult population) (Al-Janabi, Flynn, and Coast 2012); and ICECAP-SCM (a supportive care measure for use at the end of life) (Sutton and Coast 2013). As a first step in developing the ICECAP-O, researchers (Grewal et al. 2006) conducted qualitative work with older people to identify important areas of life. The data suggested that quality of life of respondents was affected by losing the ability to pursue the things they valued and so the five areas of life identified were interpreted as capabilities (Coast et al. 2008a; Grewal et al. 2006), see Table 1.

For each question, there are four levels of capability and the respondent can choose one, for example: "I can have all of the love and friendship that I want." Levels below this are "a lot," "a little" and "cannot have any." What is essentially being assessed is whether the respondent judges that they are free and able to function at the level at which they desire. The authors therefore refer to "perceived capability" (Coast et al. 2008a). A degree of subjectivity is therefore introduced over and above that which might be associated with simple reporting of the level of functioning.

The ICECAP-A (Al-Janabi, Flynn, and Coast 2012) and ICECAP-SCM (Sutton and Coast 2013) were similarly developed and have five and seven dimensions, respectively.

Table 1. Summary of capability measures

Nussbaum's central capabilities	WHODAS 2.0	ICECAP-A	ICECAP-O	Assessment of capability in patients with chronic pain	Ruger's health capability paradigm
Life	Cognition	Stability	Attachment	Love and social inclusion	Different applications will require different measures, but broadly, the health capability profile will contain information on health functioning and health agency
Bodily health	Mobility	Attachment	Security	Enjoyment	
Bodily integrity	Self-care	Autonomy	Role	Respect and identity	
Senses, imagination and thought	Getting along (interacting with other people)	Achievement	Enjoyment	Remaining physically and mentally active	*Health functioning:* could be assessed using instruments such as SF-36, biomarkers or the presence of risk factors
Emotions	Life activities	Enjoyment	Control	Societal and family roles	
Practical reason	Participation			Independence and autonomy	*Health agency:* will be determined by internal factors (such as health knowledge, motivation, values and skills) and external factors (such as social norms, political and economic circumstances and the provision of public health services)
Affiliation				Physical and mental well-being	
Species				Feeling secure about the future	
Play					
Control over one's environment					

What distinguishes the ICECAP-A from the ICECAP-O is a subtle change of wording from, for example, "I can have all of the love and friendship *that I want*" in the case of ICECAP-O, to "I can have *a lot* of love, friendship and support" in the case of ICECAP-A (emphasis added). ICECAP-SCM is different again in the respect that attribute levels are phrased in terms of time, for example, "I can make decisions that I need to make about my life and care most of the time;" this decision appears to have been influenced more by the type of attributes (which relate more closely to the processes and nature of the care being received).

Assessing capability in patients with chronic pain. A second example of the use of participatory methods focuses on chronic pain (Kinghorn 2010). Qualitative work was conducted in order to identify capabilities important to patients with chronic pain. These capabilities were developed into a questionnaire, which was piloted with a separate sample of patients (also with chronic pain) and has since been subjected to further refinement.

The work by Kinghorn (2010) still relies on self-reporting by the respondent, but (in the original version) ability/freedom in terms of higher order capabilities is assessed in terms of achievement on a number of more basic capabilities and functionings. In other words, functionings and basic capabilities are used as a proxy for the higher order capability. Although there is a danger that assessing functionings and basic capabilities will fail to incorporate all of the person's individual priorities and circumstances in respect to the higher order capability, the "proxy" measurement has legitimacy in the sense that the link between the higher order capability and the functionings/basic capabilities was identified from the qualitative work.

One unfortunate implication is that a large number of questions are needed to assess each higher order capability, hence placing greater burden on respondents. High numbers of incomplete questionnaires were returned in the pilot study, in comparison to the number of EQ-5D questionnaires returned incomplete (Kinghorn 2010). The refined version (Kinghorn, Robinson and Smith 2015) of the questionnaire (see Table 1) was a reaction to concerns about feasibility and acceptability of use and is more in keeping with the approach taken by Coast et al., in that the refined questionnaire directly asks respondents about the higher order capabilities. In refining the questionnaire, feedback was sought from a (separate) user group of patients with chronic pain.

Valuing Objects Within the Capability Set

Ruger's Health Capability Paradigm. Ruger sees no place within her paradigm for preferences and warns that preferences may not align with health need. Ruger gives the example that "in some cultures, devaluation of women might diminish preferences for maternal health during and after pregnancy" (Ruger 2009b, 59–60). Ruger's central health capabilities are valued above other non-central health capabilities in the capability set through a process of incompletely theorized agreements (Ruger 1998, 2004a, 2006a, 2006b; Ruger and Kim 2006) whereby partial ordering is combined with priority to the worst off.

The health capability profile allows for scales and subscales that can be employed by researchers and policy-makers who may want to determine weights and aggregate data across domains (Ruger 2010). Batteries of questions measuring key profile constructs were developed for studies in Vietnam (Nguyen et al. 2012) and India (Feldman et al. 2014) and the health capability paradigm has been employed for empirical medical and health systems research in low- and middle-income countries (Pratt et al. 2013; Pratt and Hyder 2015).

OxCAP instruments. Equal weight was assigned to each of the dimensions on the OxCAP-MH (as with earlier OCAP/OxCAP instruments), and individual levels are merely scored from 1 (meaning very severe limitation) to 5 (meaning no limitation) (Simon et al. 2013). The justification relates to a rejection of preferences: "collapsing multi-dimensional capabilities information into a single index score using preference-based valuation techniques is conceptually in tension with the original capability approach" (Simon et al. 2013, 195). However, there is also acknowledgement that without weighting, the instrument is unlikely to be adopted as the sole outcome measure, but is more likely to be used to provide supplementary information to decision-makers, who will rely primarily on the existing QALY framework.

ICECAP instruments. Weights reflecting the relative importance of capabilities incorporated within the ICECAP instruments have been elicited using best–worst attribute scaling (Coast et al. 2008a; Flynn, Louviere, and Coast 2007). Coast et al. acknowledge that whilst there is no suggestion in Sen's writings of a practical method for eliciting relative values for capabilities, what is explicitly clear is the rejection of choices and desire. Best–worst scaling is therefore adopted in the case of the ICECAP-O on the justification that values and not preferences are elicited (individuals are not asked to trade one thing for another) (Coast et al. 2008a).

Sen appears more critical of the adoption of utility as the evaluative space than of the use of utility-type information as an indication of an object's value, stating that: "Sometimes it might make sense to use utility-type information about strength of desire as reflecting valuation, even though the two are neither identical, nor invariably closely related to each other" (Sen 1999a, 32). Sen is careful to distinguish between the possible practical need for information relating to the implied value of an object and the adoption of utility-type variables as the foundation for evaluation/analysis. Note also my use of the term "more critical" above in relation to utility as the object of value. There is no suggestion here that Sen has endorsed any role for utility information; instead, the use of utility information as an imperfect indication of the relative value of different attributes is probably the lesser of two evils.

Like Ruger before, Coast et al. adopted the stance that life is a prerequisite for other capabilities, and hence the absence of life is equivalent to the absence of capability. Having no capability at all is anchored at zero on the scale and hence the state of dead also has a zero value.

Assessing capability in patients with chronic pain. In the case of the work focusing on chronic pain, swing-weighting was explored as a method for weighting the capabilities in the original version of the instrument (Kinghorn 2010), also because this is a choiceless approach. The valuation task was completed by members of the general public in small groups so that there was scope for discussion and deliberation to influence responses, in line with Sen's suggestion that values be arrived at via a process of "reasoned consensus," requiring public discussion and democratic understanding and acceptance (Sen 1999b, 78–79).

The capability for physical and mental well-being (from the original instrument) is treated as a central capability by Kinghorn (2010), in response to empirical data and qualitative feedback from respondents completing the swing-weighting exercise. Although valuation was only explored through a small-scale pilot study, a functional form was proposed such that having *no* capability in terms of physical and mental well-being would reduce the overall well-being score to zero, acknowledging the catastrophic affect that severe impairment to physical and mental well-being has on life. It was not deemed necessary to set the lower anchor of the scale as dead, but it follows logically that dead would have a score of zero.

Decision-making

There are two uncertainties associated with pluralist frameworks such as the CA. First, how to identify those least advantaged, the so-called "indexing problem" (Riddle 2010; Wolff and De-Shalit 2007). Second, who should be prioritized and according to what justification? In the case of the ICECAP measures, preference-type information, aggregated at a societal level, is used to create a common index in which there is an explicit relative weighting of the component capabilities. This makes a complete ordering of states possible. In the case of the ICECAP instruments, consideration as to which decision-rule to adopt (in respect to the case for redistributing resources) has been initiated as a separate project (Mitchell et al. 2015). Mitchell et al. explored the impact of setting various poverty levels, or levels of sufficient capability, and using this to adjust the anchoring of the existing scale for ICECAP, such that zero is still equivalent to no capability, but one becomes equal to "sufficient capability." In this way, priority is given to the enhancement of capability for those below the poverty level.

Kinghorn et al. explored the elicitation of relative values, although there is no suggestion as to how values would be used by decision-makers. In the case of OXCAP-MH, influence is likely to be limited to supplementing QALY information with something broader and disaggregated.

Equity is a central principle of the health capability paradigm and shortfall sufficiency is used to determine need/priority, for which a partial ordering of health capabilities and/or health functionings is all that is needed. Under Ruger's system (2009a, 269):

> priority goes to individuals who exhibit a gap between their health status and the status they could achieve, and those with the greatest deficit in health status should receive the highest priority. Priority is placed on all deprivations below the shortfall equity norm.

Ruger stresses the importance of human diversity, and it is acknowledged that, in some cases, the objective of health policy should be to bring people as close to good functioning as their natural circumstances permit (Ruger 2009b, 90). Whilst a disabled person cannot be given the freedom to enjoy the same level of functioning as a non-disabled person, there is, nevertheless, a case for maximizing his functioning ability in order to reduce the shortfall (Ruger 2009b, 92).

Ruger selects her central health capabilities on the basis that they will attract support across society as an absolute minimal acceptable threshold. Therefore, the minimum obligation to society is to ensure that no person's central health capabilities are threatened. The absolute constraint on redistribution will be the point where additional redistribution would require an individual to sacrifice her central health capabilities for the benefit of another. In other words, redistribution will occur at some level within the range in which sacrifices can be made outside of the realm of central health capabilities. The market can play a role in prioritizing non-central capabilities:

> Meeting the health needs and health agency deficits associated with central health capabilities … must precede addressing other health capabilities; the selection and weights among non-central health capabilities can await further specification … through social agreement at the next stage. (Ruger 2009b, 76)

In addition to equity, Ruger also sees efficiency as an important consideration (Ruger 2009b), although it should be noted that in the health capability paradigm, efficiency principles are applied to equity goals. The process would work as follows (Ruger 2009b, 95):

> A stepwise approach first addresses equity, using clinical input to promote equality in individuals' ability to be healthy; then it addresses efficiency by using cost-minimization analysis and, in specific cases, cost effectiveness analysis as economic input in the decision-making process.

Resources would therefore be used efficiently to enhance the capability of those deemed to be "in need" rather than being used to bring about the greatest overall increase in societal welfare.

A Critique of Interpretations of the CA Within Health

The Objective, as Reflected by the Breadth of the Capability Set

Perhaps the most notable conceptual difference when comparing these four approaches is between the stance in which health has intrinsic value (here, the capability of importance is the capability to enjoy good health), and the stance in which health is of importance both as one element of well-being and as a determinant of an individual's broader capability set. Both stances fully recognize and highlight the importance of health, so does it matter whether we treat health as the end goal or as a means to an end? In her book, *Health and Social Justice*, Ruger refers to the failure of healthcare reform in the USA and to the case of many other countries throughout the world. Indeed, the special Rapporteur on the international right to health has put forth the health capability paradigm as a possible theoretical grounding for the right to health. Ruger's motivation for outlining a core view of health—a "view from everywhere"—needs to be understood against the backdrop of a lack of consensus on moral norms relating to distributive justice and the need for a provincial and global consensus on health morality for global health justice and governance (2009b, 14).

In contrast, the three alternative interpretations have developed within the UK, a country which boasts the world's largest publicly funded healthcare service. One reason why the CA has attracted interest in the UK is the interaction between health and social care and recognition that frameworks such as the QALY (which adopt health and the healthcare sector as their sole focus) are of limited relevance when evaluating social care (as they will undervalue the impact of these services, which have a broader impact on well-being). For this reason, the National Institute for Health and Care Excellence (NICE) in the UK has recently included the use of capability instruments such as ICECAP into its guidelines for evaluating social care (NICE 2013). The concern here is twofold, the significant risk of viewing all human problems as medical problems to be addressed by the healthcare system, and the risk of undervaluing the ways in which health and social care impact upon the lives of service users. Ruger addresses this theoretically (Ruger 2004b; Ruger and Kim 2006) and empirically (Nguyen et al. 2012), for example, with health capabilities as part of the broader set of capabilities in resource allocation.

Health as the Sole Objective

With its focus on achieving health outcomes (health functioning and mortality), the health capability paradigm aligns with the QALY, but extends beyond it to include health agency. This requires the policy-maker to look "up-stream" at those factors contributing to health functioning. Factors influencing health agency may originate from the health and non-health sectors. The health capability paradigm therefore seeks to extend what is incorporated into QALYs by considering the ability to pursue health, as well as assessing health outcomes. Indeed, by incorporating the availability of information and guidance, access to health care and the existence of preventative interventions the paradigm would appear to encompass many of the same objectives as would define a public health agenda.

Whereas Ruger suggests tangible measures (such as SF-36) for the assessment of health functioning, other concepts, such as "health knowledge" could also employ existing measures or rely on the development of new ones; guidance here is not as clearly defined. The health capability paradigm is a high-level concept with a range of proposals and research to translate it into practical guidance (Feldman et al. 2014; Nguyen et al. 2012; Ruger and Kim 2006; Ruger 2010, 2012).

In terms of sectoral and budgetary considerations, there is an important difference between health capability and extra-welfarism (despite both assuming that health has intrinsic value as a merit good). The health capability paradigm is concerned with evaluating policies, interventions and societal norms in terms of their impact upon a set of health capabilities, deemed to be of special importance. The area of government responsible for initiating the policy appears to be largely irrelevant (for example, health improvement could be driven as much through improvements in literacy as through improvements in emergency medicine). In contrast, the QALY is a framework for assessing efficiency within a single sector. This adds a level of complexity to Ruger's approach which is not required by extra-welfarism. It also means, however, that the QALY places a concentrated responsibility on the health system which is not as rigidly imposed within the health capability paradigm, or indeed by those approaches which see the goal as improvements to a broad capability set.

What the QALY and the health capability paradigm share is the stance that deficiencies in health cannot be compensated for through expansions elsewhere in the capability set (Coast 2009). Indeed, Ruger states that "society should avert or ameliorate loss in physical or mental functioning even if opportunities of employment, careers, talents, or education remain possible" (Ruger 2009b, 140).

Finding a Place for Health Within the Broader Capability Set?

In the OCAP/OxCAP instruments and in work conducted by Kinghorn, health dimensions and the capability to have good physical and mental well-being (respectively) are of importance among a broad range of other capabilities/dimensions. In the ICECAP-O and A, there are no dimensions directly related to health. It is noted (Grewal et al. 2006) that "good health appeared to facilitate the ability [of participants] to do activities, and thus obtain the benefits that activities can give," (1895) that is, enjoyment, attachment and so on. It is likely that health features more prominently and independently in the work by Kinghorn because patients with chronic pain were sampled who were aware that chronic pain was the focus of the study. In the case of the OCAP/OxCAP work, capabilities such as bodily health are included within Nussbaum's central capabilities (Nussbaum 2003).

It is not clear whether, by incorporating health/physical and mental well-being, there is some degree of double counting in the OCAP/OxCAP instruments and by Kinghorn, or whether by omitting any direct reference to health there is a gap in the ICECAP-O/A. Participants in the study by Kinghorn did speak of how their pain restricted their ability to be and do the things they valued, but pain itself is also, by definition "an unpleasant sensory and emotional experience" (Coniam and Diamond 1994, 2) and is, in its own right, "attention seeking." Hence, those with serious ill health experience *both* the immediate symptoms and the subsequent impact on broader aspects of life.

It is common for the ICECAP instruments to be administered alongside a health-related instrument, but not clear how, or indeed if, data relating to health-related functionings should be considered alongside broader capability well-being. Davis et al. (2012) included ICECAP-O alongside EQ-5D-3L in the context of a falls prevention programme in Vancouver. They used exploratory factor analysis to ascertain whether the two instruments can be classed as complements or substitutes. The authors report that most of the attributes of EQ-5D load primarily onto a factor interpreted as "physical functioning," whereas most of the attributes of ICECAP-O load primarily onto a factor interpreted as "psychosocial well-being." The authors therefore conclude that ICECAP-O provides different/complimentary information to EQ-5D. If the ICECAP instruments are to be used alongside assessments of physical health-related functioning, it is not appropriate for ICECAP to duplicate the assessment of health-related functioning.

It would, however, be more accurate to view Davis et al.'s notions of physical functioning and psychosocial well-being not as separate, unrelated constructs but instead as two levels within the same hierarchical framework. The normative stance of those adopting capability as an expansionist approach is that a broad concept of well-being, defined in terms of capability, is the appropriate end point of importance. Including instruments which assess physical functioning alongside expansionist frameworks such as ICECAP fundamentally redefines the end point (or evaluative space) to one which is arbitrarily inclusive. The fact that we can capture sets of outcomes which are subtly different to those outcomes which define our intended starting point does n't mean that we should. If we did, then where would we draw the line? Perhaps there is a need then for those advocating expansionist approaches to better justify and defend the parameters of their intended evaluative space as a set of broad capabilities which are not exclusively health-related.

The question then remains that of whether health appears at the top of the hierarchy, within our set of broad capabilities of "ultimate importance" or is merely a factor influencing what is ultimately important, or indeed both. This leads back to uncertainty around the definition of health. Take, as an example, the WHODAS 2.0 (summarized in Table 1), formulated as a "standardized method for measuring health and disability" (Üstün et al. 2010, v); it does not itself directly include pain, discomfort or depression. Both the WHODAS attributes and individual items either overlap with or align closely to attributes on the ICECAP measures, and so if health is understood in this way, it would be very difficult to argue that health is missing from ICECAP. Those aspects of health included within the OCAP/OxCAP instruments and by Kinghorn relate to life expectancy and symptoms likely to be immediately attention seeking, such as pain, physical discomfort and depression. The interpretation here is not, for example, just that one's pain impacts upon one's well-being, but that one lives with the presence of pain *and* its broader impact on well-being.

Why introduce greater complexity by broadening the focus of the evaluative space beyond health? Consider a patient with chronic pain; in many cases, there will be no treatable cause for a patient's pain and the intent for that patient's care is to control symptoms and enable as close to normal functioning as possible. The same would equally apply in the example of the disabled person, used by Sen and Ruger. Given the limited (but still important) scope for medicine to improve the well-being of either of these patients, the physical, legal and cultural environments of the two patients become more relevant as conversion factors enabling or denying a good life in the broadest sense. It could be argued that there is conflict here with Ruger's position if expansion in the broader capability set is permitted as compensation for avoidable deficiencies in the provision of health. Ruger's health capability paradigm recognizes the distinctively intrinsic and interrelated joint importance of health capabilities.

When health is adopted as the end point, there is flexibility as to how to promote health and considerations may include financial cost, technology and feasibility. When broad well-being is the end point, there is flexibility as to whether to prioritize health as a means of promoting well-being and it is this flexibility that Ruger intentionally seeks to avoid. Extra-welfarism similarly does not provide scope for the health system to promote anything other than health improvement. There is no suggestion, however, that those expansionist approaches, adopting a broad capability set, would advocate any denial of feasible treatment aimed at preventing or curing a medical condition, but rather they allow for other services to "pick up the baton" when medicine reaches its current limits (or society reaches the limit of what is affordable). Is the lack of protection for health as an intrinsic good a weakness of those approaches seeking to expand the evaluative space? It may appear ironic that evaluative frameworks established with the intention of better capturing outcomes from existing health services could lead to dilution of or disinvestment in those very services, but let us remember that the resources used to produce health care are scarce. It may be as harmful to forbid any consideration of those resources being used positively elsewhere in order to achieve an expansion of well-being clearly defined, as to fail to recognize the importance of health and health care. A lack of commitment to the universal provision of adequate health care will damage well-being precisely because of the importance and magnitude of the impact of health and so broadening our evaluative space beyond health certainly does not give charter for reckless underinvestment in health care.

Expert Versus Participatory

Whilst two of the interpretations rely on expert definition of the capability set (the OxCAP and health capability paradigm), participatory methods have informed to some extent all four approaches and entirely underpin the ICECAP instruments and work on chronic pain. The natural evolution of the OCAP/OxCAP instruments at least partly explains the fact that they are expert-led—they were developed from previous exploratory work by Anand et al., which in turn was based upon Nussbaum's central capabilities. In the health capability paradigm, the evaluative space is deliberately defined so as to seek an incompletely theorized agreement. Development of ICECAP instruments and the work with chronic pain patients was intended to reflect the priorities of service users. A participatory approach has been defended by Clark, who states that: "while the poor and disadvantage[d] often report high levels of happiness and life satisfaction … they are still capable of imagining, articulating and demanding a substantially better or 'good' form of life" (Clark 2009, 26). Research cited by Clark (2009, 32) found that 90% of people who had no access to health care during their last serious illness still thought that a clinic, public hospital or better was necessary for a person to get by. Clark also warns of the risk that adaptation (real or not) is used to "justify and privilege elitist conceptions of well-being" (35).

Self-reported Functionings Versus Self-perceived Capability

It has been suggested that it will be impossible to directly assess capability (Alkire 2002; Sen 1999b) and in studies relating to human development, observed functionings tend to be used as a proxy for capability (Gasper 2007). However, a crucial difference is that in studies of human development, it is often macro-level or panel data which are analysed, whereas in health care, there is an established culture of collecting patient-level data. Coast et al. argue that the idea of a third party objectively assessing complex capabilities that include an internal element (such as attachment or security) "seems unsound" (Coast et al. 2008a, 881).

By asking about a respondent's freedom to function, rather than the level at which they *actually* function, it could be argued that the questions are respectful of the fact that individuals are likely to want to live their lives in different ways and have different priorities. There is some encouraging evidence (Al-Janabi et al. 2013) that respondents can interpret questions framed in terms of capability, as intended by the researcher, although in the study by Al-Janabi et al. a minority did find the task cognitively demanding. It can therefore tentatively be suggested that the adoption of a capability style of questioning does "add value" (additional information) compared to a more straightforward focus on functioning.

Exploiting a cluster-randomized controlled trial of a community-based behaviour change management intervention in India, researchers studying health agency focused on participant "abilities" (for example, ability to obtain health education or to make independent decisions) as well as "perceived abilities" (Feldman et al. 2014).

Unless it is shown that different groups systematically interpret the phrasing of questions in terms of capability in different ways, then asking for self-reported capability may be no less problematic than asking about self-reported health functioning. Sen, for example, illustrates how self-reported levels of health can provide contradictory evidence to actual life expectancy and suggests that factors such as literacy and living conditions influence self-reporting of health (Sen 2002).

Decision-making

Both Ruger and Mitchell et al. have proposed some form of sufficiency, although seemingly (again) with different interpretations. Ruger's proposal for partial ordering and shortfall sufficiency rely on a crucial assumption/simplification, namely that central health capabilities can be defined transpositionally with widespread support. A deficiency in terms of central health capabilities would constitute a shortfall and trigger support through redistribution. But has Ruger succeeded in defining a concept of health which can reflect the view from everywhere? It is one thing to gain consensus in relation to the definition of two central health capabilities (avoiding premature death and escapable mortality); it is another to gain consensus in terms of the observable data on health functionings that should be adopted as a proxy for those health capabilities, and what level of detriment in relation to any one specific functioning is tolerated before the individual is deemed to drop below the threshold level. Ruger has conducted ethical and empirical work on premature mortality, employing observable data on adult and child mortality to define, through cluster analytical techniques, a global norm or threshold of achievable health (Ruger and Kim 2006).

The instruments which Ruger suggests should be used (such as SF-36 or other measures of physical, mental and social functioning) were not developed to reflect any form of consensus on what are deemed to be central aspects of health. It is not obvious that having "some limitations" in terms of strenuous sports and heavy lifting (an item from the SF-36) is accepted as an objective global indicator of escapable morbidity. Few respondents completing such measures would be found to have no limitations whatsoever, and so some cut-off *will* be required (given that resources are finite). Hence, whilst shortfall sufficiency is the only contender which can be identified from the four approaches considered in this paper, and whilst it is undoubtedly conceptually appealing, there will still be a level of value judgement involved with operationalizing it.

Ruger has advanced theoretical and empirical work on premature death, one of the central health capabilities, and applied it to better understanding theoretical levels of adult and child mortality as ethically and empirically relevant cut-offs. Her paradigm then employs efficiency analysis to assess the limits of domestic and global obligations.

Where Next?

Health: A Means or an End?

Whether one embarks upon an assessment of the capability to experience good health or an assessment of a broader capability set, influenced by health and social care systems, is likely to depend upon the policy question and the context. Whilst focus on a core concept of health may be useful for driving healthcare reform, or indeed for comparing and benchmarking the progress of different health systems, the merit of adopting a sole focus on health when planning resource allocation at a (relatively) local decision-making level is increasingly being questioned in countries such as the UK.

If the health capability paradigm is to be distinguished from QALYs in a workable form, then there is a need for greater direction from Ruger as to how health agency (rather than simply health functioning) should be assessed. It is difficult to see how health agency could be assessed without an examination of certain characteristics of a health system and this may mean that overall (i.e. when combined with health functioning), the health capability paradigm relies on the interpretation of a wide, complex and disaggregated array of information. Conceptual and empirical approaches have been advanced to operationalize the health capability paradigm (Feldman et al. 2014; Nguyen et al. 2012; Ruger and Kim 2006; Ruger 2010, 2012).

The inclusion of the ICECAP instruments within NICE guidance in the UK is a significant breakthrough for the CA in health economics, but is far from being an end point as more methodological work is still needed. If adopting the normative stance that health should be evaluated—at least in part—through its influence on a broad capability set, then it may be unacceptable to use the same capability set to assess the well-being of every individual in the population. Instead, the assessment should respect the fact that at different stages of life, we experience different levels of dependency and vulnerability, and we fulfil different roles within the family and wider society. Hence, as an initial and tentative suggestion, a different capability set may be needed for children, adults, those with severe cognitive impairment and those in the last few weeks or days of life.

I would argue, consistent with Ruger (2010), that health should be understood, to some extent, as an end as well as a means. There may be some argument for protecting and acknowledging the special importance of health and so "weighting the balance" of evaluative frameworks to favour health—essentially accepting the risk of double counting. I would, however, be influenced more by the accounts of the patients with chronic pain who spoke of and displayed signs that their pain demanded their immediate attention as an unpleasant sensory emotion. Just as a rejection of happiness as the sole indicator of well-being does not lead Sen to entirely exclude happiness from his concept of well-being, so it may be wrong to exclude any careful consideration of health in response to a rejection of health as the entire evaluative space.

I believe (and I refer back to Clark's work, as well as to related standpoint theory; Wylie 2003, in order to justify such a position) that there is a role for identifying important capabilities through participatory work. Given the suggestion to differentiate instruments based upon broad population groupings, and given the striking similarity between capabilities identified from such broad population groups (as with ICECAP) and those identified as important to specific patient groups (as done by Kinghorn in the case of chronic pain), a proliferation of "condition specific" measures is unlikely to be a productive focus for future research.

Valuation of Objects Within the Capability Set

Whilst Ruger predicts a need for iterative partial ordering, the fact that instruments such as ICECAP have been valued using techniques such as best–worst scaling means that we have evidence as to the relative value of those capabilities defined within the instrument and the perceived severity of detriments in the levels of those capabilities. The choice of valuation technique by those developing the ICECAP instruments and indeed any process for valuing capabilities is not widely supported by those working in this area, and the exact nature of the values (preference or non-preference) is debateable. What we are yet to understand is the relative value of health versus not directly health-related capabilities/functionings. It may be, as the very preliminary findings by Kinghorn (2010) suggested, that health is a capability of central importance. It would appear intuitively correct that as individuals, we value a broader set of capabilities only if we are experiencing some level of health which is not catastrophically restrictive and distressing.

However, even a complete ordering of capability states is still not sufficient to inform selection of the shortfall threshold (if this is the decision-rule adopted), which would also need to be informed by epidemiology, expected expenditure, planned budgets and political debate. If different capability sets are developed for those at different stages of life, this will add further complexity in terms of setting a threshold. There is (possibly an essential) role for valuation, but future debate and research should look at what it means to arrive at such values through "reasoned consensus."

Decision-making

Adoption of shortfall sufficiency would result in a significant policy and research shift away from the evaluation of new health technologies according to their efficiency and towards indicating which patient groups, conditions and health effects are to be prioritized. This is because efficiency is the second step, after equity and equity relies on identifying those with a legitimate shortfall. It would be natural for pharmaceutical research to follow trends in terms of where those shortfalls are identified. This may limit the development of treatments which effectively enhance "health" in controversial clinical areas deemed by society to be futile. It may also result in a greater allocation of resources to currently controversial areas such as rare (or "orphan") diseases, with a smaller proportion of the population receiving a greater share of health spending.

Setting a shortfall threshold which does not bankrupt society and against which improvement can be meaningfully judged may also require the instruments with which capability is assessed to have greater sensitivity to change within each dimension (or, put another way, to have greater power to discriminate between individuals in society).

Shortfall sufficiency is given monopoly-like status here because it is the only real suggestion found within any of the four interpretations of capability which have been considered, but (as stressed above) its adoption would have a significant impact on the policy landscape and on the academic and pharmaceutical research agendas; the possible impact needs to be explored, as well as any alternatives.

Disclosure Statement

No potential conflict of interest was reported by the author.

Note

1. The QALY is used by health technology assessment agencies in the UK, Canada and Australia. The EuroQoL group (the developers of and promoters of research into the EQ-5D, commonly used as the basis for QALYs)

was founded by researchers across England, Finland, The Netherlands, Norway and Sweden, and has since expanded.

References

Al-Janabi, H., T. Flynn, and J. Coast. 2012. "Development of a Self-report Measure of Capability Wellbeing for Adults: The ICECAP-A." *Quality of Life Research* 21 (1): 167–176.

Al-Janabi, H., T. Keeley, P. Mitchell, and J. Coast. 2013. "Can Capabilities be Self-reported? A Think Aloud Study." *Social Science & Medicine* 87: 116–122.

Alkire, S. 2002. *Valuing Freedoms. Sen's Capability Approach and Poverty Reduction*. New York: Oxford University Press.

Anand, P. 2005. "Capabilities and Health." *Journal of Medical Ethics* 31: 299–303.

Anand, P., G. Hunter, and R. Smith. 2005. "Capabilities and Well-being: Evidence Based on the Sen-Nussbaum Approach to Welfare." *Social Indicators Research* 74 (1): 9–55.

Broome, J. 2000. "Cost–Benefit Analysis and Population." In *Cost–Benefit Analysis: Legal, Economic and Philosophical Perspectives*, edited by M. D. Adler and E. A. Posner, 117–134. Chicago, IL: The University of Chicago Press.

Brouwer, W., A. J. Culyer, N. J. van Exel, and F. F. H. Rutten. 2008. "Welfarism Vs. Extra-welfarism." *Journal of Health Economics* 27: 325–338.

Clark, D. A. 2009. "Adaptation, Poverty and Well-being: Some Issues and Observations with Special Reference to the Capability Approach and Development Studies." *Journal of Human Development and Capabilities* 10 (1): 21–42.

Coast, J. 2009. "Maximisation in Extra-welfarism: A Critique of the Current Position in Health Economics." *Social Science & Medicine* 69: 786–792.

Coast, J., T. Flynn, L. Natarajan, K. Sproston, J. Lewis, J. J. Louviere, and T. J. Peters. 2008. "Valuing the ICECAP Capability Index for Older People." *Social Science & Medicine* 67: 874–882.

Coast, J., R. D. Smith, and P. Lorgelly. 2008a. "The Influence of Capabilities on Health Care Decision Making in the UK." *Social Science & Medicine* 67: 1190–1198.

Coast, J., R. D. Smith, and P. Lorgelly. 2008b. "Should the Capability Approach Be Applied in Health Economics?" *Health Economics* 17: 667–670.

Coniam, S. W., and A. W. Diamond. 1994. *Practical Pain Management*. Oxford: Oxford Medical Publications.

Cookson, R. 2005. "QALYs, and the Capability Approach." *Health Economics* 14 (8): 817–829.

Culyer, A. J. 1991. "The Normative Economics of Health Care Finance and Provision." In: *Providing Healthcare: The Economics of Alternative Systems of Finance and Delivery*, edited by A. McGuire, P. Fenn and K. Mayhew, 65–98. Oxford: Oxford University Press.

Davis, J. C., T. Liu-Ambrose, C. G. Richardson, and S. Bryan. 2012. "A Comparison of the ICECAP-O with EQ-5D in a Falls Prevention Clinical Setting: Are They Complements or Substitutes?" *Quality of Life Research*. doi:10.1007/s11136–012-0225-4

Feldman, C. H., G. L. Darmstadt, V. Kumar, and J. P. Ruger. 2014. "Women's Political Participation and Health: A Health Capability Study in Rural India." *Journal of Health Politics, Policy & Law*. doi:10.1215/03616878-2854621

Flynn, T., J. J. Louviere, and J. Coast. 2007. "Best–Worst Scaling: What It Can Do for Health Care Research and How To Do It." *Journal of Health Economics* 26: 171–189.

Gasper, D. 2007. "What Is the Capability Approach? Its Core, Rationale, Partners and Dangers." *Journal of Socio-Economics* 36: 335–359.

Grewal, I., J. Lewis, J. Brown, J. Bond, and J. Coast. 2006. "Developing Attributes for a Generic Quality of Life Measure for Older People: Preferences or Capabilities?" *Social Science & Medicine* 62: 1891–1901.

Kinghorn, P. 2010. "Developing a Capability Approach to Measure and Value Quality of Life: An Application to Chronic Pain." PhD thesis, School of Medicine, Health Policy & Practice, University of East Anglia.

Kinghorn, P., A. Robinson, and R. D. Smith. 2015. "Developing a Capability-Based Questionnaire as an Alternative Method for Assessing Well-Being in Patients with Chronic Pain." *Social Indicators Research* 120: 897–916.

Lorgelly, P., K. Lorimer, E. Fenwick, and A. Briggs. 2008. *The Capability Approach: Developing an Instrument for Evaluating Public Health Interventions*. Glasgow: University of Glasgow.

Mitchell, P., T. E. Roberts, P. M. Barton, and J. Coast. 2015. "Assessing Sufficient Capability: A New Approach to Economic Evaluation." *Social Science & Medicine* 139: 71–79.

Morris, S., N. Devlin, and D. Parkin. 2007. *Economic Analysis in Health Care*. Chichester: Wiley.

Nguyen, K., O. Khuat, C. Pham, and J. P. Ruger. 2012. "Impact of Health Insurance on Health Care Treatment and Cost in Vietnam: A Health Capability Approach to Financial Protection." *American Journal of Public Health* 102 (8): 1450–1461.

NICE. 2013. "The Social Care Guidance Manual." Accessed November 5, 2014. https://www.nice.org.uk/article/pmg10/resources/non-guidance-the-social-care-guidance-manual-pdf.

Nussbaum, M. C. 2003. "Capabilities as Fundamental Entitlements: Sen and Social Justice." *Feminist Economics* 9 (2–3): 33–59.

Pratt, B., and A. Hyder. 2015. "Applying a Global Justice Lens to Health Systems Research Ethics: An Initial Exploration." *Kennedy Institute of Ethics Journal* 25 (1): 35–66.

Pratt, B., D. Zion, P. Y. Cheah, F. Nosten, and B. Loff. 2013. "Ancillary Care: From Theory to Practice in International Clinical Research." *Public Health Ethics* 6 (2): 154–169.

Riddle, C. 2010. "Indexing, Capabilities, and Disability." *Journal of Social Philosophy* 41 (4): 527–537.

Robeyns, I. 2006. "The Capability Approach in Practice*." *The Journal of Political Philosophy* 14 (3): 351–376.

Ruger, J. P. 1998. "Aristotelian Justice and Health Policy: Capability and Incapacity Theorized Agreements." PhD diss., Harvard University.

Ruger, J. P. 2004a. "Health and Social Justice." *The Lancet* 364: 1075–1080.

Ruger, J. P. 2004b. "Ethics of the Social Determinants of Health." *The Lancet* 364 (9439): 1092–1097.

Ruger, J. P. 2006a. "Measuring Disparities in Health Care." *British Medical Journal* 333 (7562): 274.

Ruger, J. P. 2006b. "Toward a Theory of a Right to Health: Capability and Incompletely Theorized Agreements." *Yale Journal of Law and Humanities* 18 (2): 273–326.

Ruger, J. P. 2009a. "Global Health Justice." *Public Health Ethics* 2 (3): 261–275.

Ruger, J. P. 2009b. *Health and Social Justice*. New York: Oxford University Press.

Ruger, J. P. 2010. "Health Capability: Conceptualization and Operationalization." *American Journal of Public Health* 100 (1): 41–49.

Ruger, J. P. 2012. "An Alternative Framework for Analysing Financial Protection in Health." *PLoS Medicine* 9 (8): e1001294.

Ruger, J. P., and H. J. Kim. 2006. "Global Health Inequalities: An International Comparison." *Journal of Epidemiology and Community Health* 60 (11): 928–936.

Saith, R. 2011. "A Public Health Perspective on the Capability Approach." *Journal of Human Development and Capabilities* 12 (4): 587–594.

Sen, A. 1999a. *Commodities and Capabilities*. New Delhi: Oxford University Press.

Sen, A. 1999b. *Development as Freedom*. New York: Oxford University Press.

Sen, A. 2002. "Health: Perception Versus Observation." *BMJ* 324: 860–861.

Simon, J., P. Anand, A. Gray, J. Rugkasa, K. Yeeles, and T. Burns. 2013. "Operationalising the Capability Approach for Outcome Measurement in Mental Health Research." *Social Science & Medicine*. doi:10.1016/j.socscimed.2013.09.019

Sutton, E., and J. Coast. 2013. "Development of a Supportive Care Measure for Economic Evaluations of End-of-life Care Using Qualitative Methods." *Palliative Medicine*. doi:10.1177/0269216313489368

Torrance, G. W. 1986. "Measurement of Health State Utilities for Economic Appraisal: A Review." *Journal of Health Economics* 5 (1): 1–30.

Üstün, T. B., N. Korstanjsek, S. Chatterji, and J. Rehm. 2010. *Measuring Health and Disability: Manual for WHO Disability Assessment Schedule*. Geneva: World Health Organisation.

Verkerk, M. A., J. J. V. Busschbach, and E. D. Karssing. 2001. "Health-related Quality of Life Research and the Capability Approach of Amartya Sen." *Quality of Life Research* 10 (1): 49–55.

WHO. 1946. *Preamble to the Constitution of the World Health Organization*. New York. Official Records of the WHO, No. 2, p. 100.

Wolff, J., and A. De-Shalit. 2007. *Disadvantage*. Oxford: Oxford University Press.

Wylie, A. 2003. *Science and Other Cultures: Issues in Philosophies of Science & Technology*. London: Routledge (R. Figueroa and S. Harding).

Index

abilities: of business partners 80; perceived 8
abuse of people with disabilities 53
Acosta, Alberto 14
adverse selection 109
Afghanistan 47, 58
Afrikaans identity 38
agency: *achieved* or *instrumental* 16; definition of 15–16, 114; freedom of 15–16; personal 15, 18; *see also* health agency
Akerlof, George 109
Alfares, H.K. 54
Al-Janabi, H. 139
Alkire, Sabina 30, 47, 50, 64, 78, 86
Allais paradox 115–16
altruistic behaviour 111
Anand, P. 130, 138
Aristotle 118
Arrow, Kenneth 108–9
aspiration 39, 42
autonony, personal 12–13, 26

Bardin, Laurence 16
Bayer CropScience 4, 76–81, 84–7
Bayes' rule 115
Becker, Gary 111
behavioural economics 112
benevolence of business partners 80
best-worst scaling 141
Biggeri, M. 47, 58
"bottomless pit" investment 123
bounded rationality 112
Burchardt, Tania 13–15, 20

Cambodia 76
Cameron, John 79
Cannings, T.I. 47, 58
capabilities: listings of 32–42; *perceived* or *self-perceived* 130, 138–9; *see also* health capabilities
capability approach (CA) 1–7, 11–16, 25–6, 29–32, 35, 42–3, 46–50, 76–81, 89–90, 114, 119, 127–41; critique of interpretation 135–40
capability sets 135–6, 140–1; definition of 129–32

Chakraborty, Rhyddhi 4
Chaouia-Ouardhiga region 48
child labor 81
Chile 2, 11–13, 16
choice functions 110–11
chronic pain 7–8, 132–3, 136–40
Clark, D.A. 138, 140
Coast, J. 132–3, 138–9
Coca-Cola (company) 3
collectivism 13–14, 25
common good 31, 116–17, 120
Coniam, S.W. 136
constitutional guarantees 32
content analysis 2, 11–13, 16–18, 23–5
context specificity 41
"conversion handicap" (Sen) 31, 64
Cookson, R. 128
cooperation, reasons for 116–17
corporate initiatives 3–4, 76, 80, 86–90
corporate social responsibility (CSR) 76
cost-effectiveness analysis 123
cost-minimization analysis 123
cost-utility analysis 127–8
Crocker, Davd 15
cultural linkage 39

Darfur 47, 58
Davis, J.C. 137
Deaton, Angus 120
decision-making 134–5, 139–41
dental health 86, 88
dependency, situations of 12–13, 18–20, 23–6
deprivation: dimensions of 3, 52; indicators of 46; overlap of 54–5; rates of 55–6
De-Shalit, A. 32, 35–41
Diamond, A.W. 136
"dilemma of difference" 31–2
disability 1–3, 123–4; costs associated with 47; definition of 11, 13, 35, 50; extent of 12; measures of 49; *medical* and *social* perspectives on 30
disability-inclusive policy for higher education 29–43
disability-screening questionnaire (DSQ) 49–50
discrimination 65

Dreze, Jean 96
Duffuaa, S.O. 54

"earning handicap" (Sen) 31, 64
education 2, 51, 64; *see also* higher education
efficiency, economic concept of 110; *see also* Pareto efficiency
Ellsberg paradox 115
employment 51, 64
equal access 121–2
equal opportunity 14
equity 134–5
Erb, S. 47
ethical issues 5, 109–10, 113–20, 124
extra-welfarism 6–8, 114–15, 128, 136, 138
Eyeson, Abena 79

fairness, sense of 117
first optimality theory of economics 108
Flanagan, Tara 13
focus group discussions (FGDs) 82–4
Folland, Sherman 109–10
food supply 84
Foster, James 47, 50, 64
freedom, *process-oriented* or *outcome-oriented* 114

game theory 113, 115
Goodman, Allen C. 109–10
"goodness" of a health state 127–8
Greenwald, B.C. 109
Grewal, I. 136
Grut, L. 47

happiness 140
Harris-White, B. 47
health 3–8; core concept of 17, 127, 140; definition 77, 100, 128, 137; as a *means to an end* or having *intrinsic value* 135–41; in Morocco and Tunisia 51, 60; *objective* and *subjective* measures of 4; right to 135; social determinants of 94, 120–1
health agency 100–2, 114, 119, 121, 124, 127–30, 135–6, 140
health capabilities 1, 4–8, 77–9, 89–90, 113, 118–20; *central* or *secondary* 119, 134, 139, 141; gaps in 79; linked to human flourishing 118–19; summary of methods of measuring of 131; swing-weighting applied to 133; of those living with disabilities 120;
Health Capability Paradigm (HCP) 1, 4–8, 94–6, 100–4, 108–10, 114–24, 127–41
health economics 108–10, 114–18, 121, 124, 127
health evaluation, *subjective* and *objective* 82–4
health governance, shared 101, 104, 121–2
health improvement 136
health inequality 78, 94–5; social construct-ion of 94
health insurance 122, 130
health perceptions, *subjective* or *objective* 84–5
health-related measures 85–6
healthcare: "bottom-up" strategy for 96; incompleteness and inconsistency of 115; private sector provision of 3; universal coverage of 103–4
herd mentality 116
higher education: disability-inclusive policy for 29–43
human capital 79
human flourishing 118–19, 122, 129
Hunter, G. 130

ICECAP instruments 7–8, 130–41
identity, choice of 40, 42
impartiality 117
independence, definition of 12
"indexing problem" 134
India 4–6, 47, 81, 94–104, 132, 139; healthcare system and health inequalities in 97–100; National Rural Health Mission (NRHM) 96; recommendations for health policy 102–4
inequity aversionn 117–18
information asymmetries 109
Ingstad, B. 47
integrity of contract partners 80
internal consistency of choice, theory of 110–11
International Classification of Function-ing, Disability and Health (ICF) 49

James, Philip 79
job opportunities 51, 64

Kahneman, Daniel 112
Kenya 47
Kinghorn, P. 7–8, 132–7, 140–1
knowledge and imagination, capability of 36

language capability 38
learning disposition 38
listings of capabiities 32–42
living conditions 53
Longelly, P. 130
low- and middle-income countries (LMIC) 46–7, 64

malaria 86
Malhotra, Deepak 80
malnutrition see nutrition and malnutrition
Marfull-Jensen, Marisol 13
marginalized groups 41
market failure 5, 109
Mauro, V. 47, 58
Merck (company) 3
Millennium Development Goals 51
Mitchell, P. 139

Mitra, Sophie (co-editor) 31, 47, 54, 58, 60
mobility within universities 40
Model Village Project (MVP) 4, 76, 79–82, 85–9
Morocco 2, 46–51, 55–60, 64–5
motivation, *instrumental* or *social* 117
multinational corporations (MNCs) 3–4, 76–82, 85–90
Mutanga, Oliver 2, 29

Nagel, Thomas 111
National Institute for Health and Care Excellence (NICE) 135, 140
neoclassical economics 5–6
Ng, Nora Y. 79
norms, moral 120, 135
Norway 113
Nussbaum, Martha 1, 7, 29, 31–2, 65, 129–30, 136, 138
nutrition and malnutrition 51, 83–4

OCAP/OxCAP instruments 7, 130, 133–8
opportunity costs 110, 123

Pareto efficiency 5–6, 108–9
participatory ranking 54
perseverance, academic 38
pesons with severe disabilities (PWSD) 16–20, 23–5
pesticides 88
pharmaceutical research 141
Pirson, Michael 80
positive economics 6
poverty 3, 12, 46–7; multidimensional nature of 47, 50–60, 64
preference 110; *see also* revealed preference
prioritization 119, 134, 141
"prisoner's dilemma" game 113
probabilities*:* *actual* or *presumed* 115; *objective* or *subjective* 115
prospect theory 112, 116
psychological well-being 53, 65, 60, 137
public-private partnerships 3

Qizilbash, Mozaffar 13
quality-adjusted life-years (QALYs) 7–8, 114–15, 119, 127, 134, 136, 140
Querejeta González, Miguel 12

Rabat-Salé region 48
randomized controlled trials 139
rare diseases 141
rationality 110–16, 120–1 narrow view of 116; *see also* bounded rationality
"reasoned consensus" 141
Reindal, S.M. 31
religion 40
resilience, educational 35–8, 42
resource allocation 128–9, 135, 138
respect, dignity and recognition, capability of 36–7, 42
revealed preference 111–12
risk, voluntary 121
Ruger, Jennifer Prah (co-editor) 14, 78–9, 82, 88–9, 100–4, 127, 129, 132–41
rural communities, 39, 58–60, 96, 99

Saith, R. 128
Salais, R. 31
"same treatment" policy, problem with 37
Samuelson, Paul A. 110
Sánchez, Natalia 26
Scanlon, Thomas M. 124
Schelling, Thomas C. 112
Schölmerich, Maike J. 76
security and insecurity, indicators of 53
self-goal choice 113
self-interest 111–14, 117
self-reported functionings 138–9
Sen, Amartya 1, 3, 11–16, 29–32, 47, 78, 82, 84, 90, 96, 100, 109–14, 128–9, 133, 137, 139
shortfall equality 119–20
shortfall inequality 95, 101, 104, 118
shortfall sufficiency 6, 8, 127, 134, 139, 141
Simon, Herbert A. 112
Slovic, Paul 112
Smith, R. 130
smoking 112
social care 135
social choice theory 119
social contract theory 31–2
social justice 31–2, 43, 50, 65, 101, 104, 112, 129
social participation 53
social relations and social networks 37, 42
social welfare functions 5, 115, 122
socialization 117
South Africa 2, 29–43
stakeholders 80
Stano, Miron 109–10
Stiglitz, Joseph E. 109
stigma 64–5
students with disabilities 29–30
sustainable development 3–4, 76–7, 85, 89
sustainable development goals (SDGs) 30

Terzi, L. 31
Trani, Jean-François 2–3, 47, 47, 58
transitivity and intransitivity 110–16
trans-positionality 119
trust: building of 85, 87; definition of 4, 79–80; organizational 80; as a prerequisite for change 79–81
Tunisia 2, 46–51, 55–60, 64–5
Tversky, Amos 112

uncertainty, conceptualization of 115

United Kingdom 135, 140
United Nations Convention on the Rights of Persons with Disabilities (CRPD) (2006) 2, 11, 14, 26, 48
United States 109, 135
University of the Free State (UFS) 34–8
University of Venda (UniVen) 34–9
Üstün, T.B. 137
utilitarianism 113–14, 123, 127
utility theory 115–16, 128

vaccination 110–11, 116
Venda community 38
Vietnam 7, 132
"voice" 41–2

Walker, M. 2, 29, 32–7, 41–2
Walters, David 79
water supply 84–6
welfare health economics 5–6
welfare maximization 112
well-being, concept of 15, 26, 113–16, 120, 133–40; freedom of 16; *see also* psychological well being
Whitehead, Margaret 94
Wilson-Strydom, M. 38
Wolff, J. 32, 35–41
women, devaluation of 64–5, 132
World Health Organization (WHO) 77, 128

Yemen 47